ASIAN CUISINES

Food Culture from East Asia to Turkey and Afghanistan

ASIAN CUISINES

Food Culture from East Asia to Turkey and Afghanistan

Edited by

Karen Christensen

Authors

**E. N. Anderson, Paul D. Buell,
Darra Goldstein,** *et al.*

BERKSHIRE
A global point of reference

Permissions may also be obtained via Copyright Clearance Center, 222 Rosewood Drive, Danvers, MA 01923, USA, telephone +1 978 750 8400, fax +1 978 646 8600, info@copyright.com.

Digital editions: *Asian Cuisines* is available through most major e-book and database services (please check with them for pricing).

For information, contact:
Berkshire Publishing Group
122 Castle Street
Great Barrington, Massachusetts 01230-1506 USA
Email: info@berkshirepublishing.com
Tel: +1 413 528 0206
Fax: +1 413 541 0076

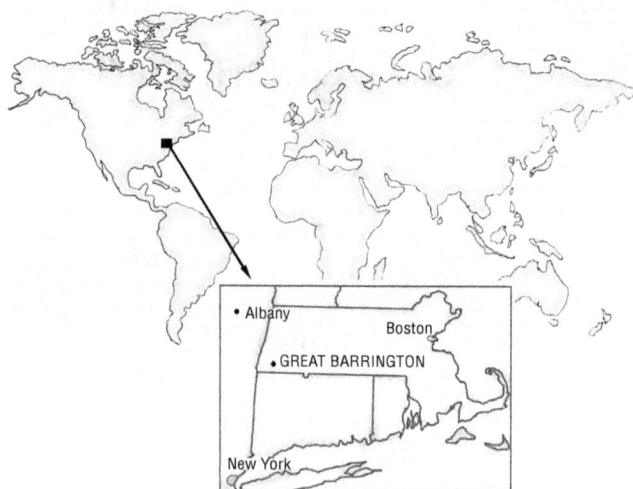

Library of Congress Cataloging-in-Publication Data

Names: Christensen, Karen, 1957- editor. | Container of (work): Anderson, E. N., 1941- China. | Container of (work): Buell, Paul D. Mongolia.
Title: Asian cuisines : food culture from East Asia to Turkey and Afghanistan / editor, Karen Christensen ; authors, E.N. Anderson, Paul Buell, et al.
Description: Great Barrington, Massachusetts : Berkshire Publishing Group, 2018. | Series: Berkshire essentials | Includes bibliographical references.
Identifiers: LCCN 2017057760| ISBN 9781614720300 (pbk. : alk. paper) | ISBN 9781614728467 (ebook)
Subjects: LCSH: Diet—Asia. | Food habits—Asia.
Classification: LCC TX360.A74 A85 2018 | DDC 394.1/2095—dc23 LC record available at https://lccn.loc.gov/2017057760

Table of Contents

Introduction

By Karen Christensen

It is hard to take in just how diverse Asia is in terms of language, religion, economy, forms of government, history, and culture. There is no single historical or modern feature that defines or unites all of Asia. There is no religion like Christianity, which has long provided unity across Europe and the New World. In Asia, Islam is the most widespread religion, but is a minority religion in several large nations such as Japan, India, China, and the Philippines; and the majority of people in Asia are not Muslims. Buddhism is the major religion in East and mainland Southeast Asia but is no longer important in Central Asia and never was in West Asia.

Western colonialism has also failed to produce regional unity as it has in parts of Africa. China has had much influence in East and northern Southeast Asia, but little in Central and West Asia. Asian colonization by the Mongols moving south and west, Hindu Indians moving east, and the Chinese moving south and east has had sub-regional rather than regional influence.

History, geography, trade, and religion have shaped the cuisines of Asia. Modern political boundaries sometimes only bear faint relation to the realities established over generations of shared traditions, rituals, and recipes.

This small volume, *Asian Cuisines: Food Culture from East Asia to Turkey and Afghanistan*, provides a succinct overview of food history, food culture, and food science across the world's largest and most diverse continent. It is unique in covering not only East, Southeast, and South Asia, but also Central Asia, the countries that straddle Asia and the Middle East, and Turkey.

Diffusion, not surprisingly, is central to the Asian gastronomic experience. A dish called Hainanese Chicken Rice, for example, may be Singaporean but is named for an island in China, and is served throughout Southeast Asia. The chili pepper is a native of the Americas but is now strongly associated with the Chinese provinces of Sichuan and Hunan, even appearing as symbolic of the rugged rural peasantry.

The realities of climate and terrain also shape culinary traditions. For example, meat and milk from herds of sheep, camels, and horses provided the basic diet of the nomadic peoples of Kazakhstan and Kyrgyzstan, while inhabitants of Tajikistan, Turkmenistan, and Uzbekistan cultivated crops and developed sophisticated cooking techniques.

It's no surprise that Indonesia, a country composed of thousands of islands, should have a cuisine as distinct and diverse as its archipelago, which has for centuries been one of the major trade routes between India, China, and the Middle East. Nor is it a surprise that the cuisines of Malaysia's three main ethnic groups—the Malays, Chinese, and Indians—form the core of Malaysian cuisine. Across much of southern and southeastern Asia, the village and family life based around wet-rice agriculture have been a powerful unifying force. In South Asia—Bangladesh, India, and Pakistan—the use of spices and sauces provides a unifying thread in otherwise diverse cuisines, as does a variety of unleavened flat breads made with wheat flour, rice, and ground legumes. One might say that Asian cuisines are first and fundamentally about fusion.

Geography plays a particularly clear role in cuisines where the Wallace line, a kind of Ice-age geological fault line, divides the Indonesian archipelago into two parts. The western part consists of the larger islands of Sumatra, Java, Bali, and Kalimantan, while the eastern part consists of Sulawesi, Maluku, the Lesser Sunda Islands, and West Papua. The distinctly different fauna and flora have led to distinctive cuisines.

In modern times, Asian nations have experienced very different patterns of economic development, with some relying on a single resource, such as oil or natural gas or timber, others on industrialized farming, others on manufacturing and others on a service-based economy. Asia contains several of the world's poorest nations (Afghanistan and Nepal), the second and third economies in the world (China and Japan), and the fastest-growing economy (China). Food supplies have frequently been a problem due to high population growth, natural disasters, and faulty economic and political policies.

Culturally and linguistically, the region is the most complex in the world. There are thousands of languages spoken across Asia and in several nations (including, for example, India, China, and Indonesia) people speak many different languages and dialects. Asia is also home to at least a thousand different cultural groups, some of whom have never been studied carefully. India and Indonesia have several hundred each, China has at least fifty-five, and even ethnically homogeneous nations such as Japan and Iran have visible ethnic minorities. This, naturally, adds to the rich, delicious complexity of Asian cuisines.

We decided to compile this collection as we became immersed in work on the five-volume *Berkshire Encyclopedia of Chinese Cuisines,* our first big food project. In our research, we discovered just how much material about food Berkshire had already published in previous reference works. The *Encyclopedia of Modern Asia*, published in 2001 in partnership with Scribner, in particular included a wealth of food-related articles with an immense geographic range. For this book, we have adapted and updated material from a number of publications and added new chapters on Iraq, Singapore, Laos, and Vietnam. In addition to covering the cuisines of different regions and specific countries, we include Pan-Asian topics such as rice, tofu, tea, and the spice trade.

It has been a pleasure to work with familiar authors again, especially E. N. Anderson and Paul D. Buell, who both graciously spent time and effort reviewing, updating, and composing new articles. We are also happy to bring new contributors into the Berkshire community, who always impress with their knowledge of and enthusiasm for their topic. Nawal Nasrallah, for example, contributed the article on Iraqi cuisine, and shared some of her favorite, and delicious, recipes. Geraldine Moreno and Carol Ireson-Doolittle submitted their article on Lao cuisine in between research trips to Asia. For some topics, finding contributors can be unexpectedly difficult, so we are delighted that Cecilia Leong-Salobir was willing to write the entry on Singapore on such short notice. Suitable recipes for Singapore, Malaysia, and Indonesia came from the personal network of our copyeditor Olette Trouve.

As the project continued, this complexity became clear to us, and we realized that perhaps the best way to better understand it, was to try out various dishes for ourselves. At Berkshire Publishing, a love of cooking and baking is the common denominator among the employees, so we were excited to start cooking. Our authors recommended their favorite recipes or dishes. We hope that many readers will have the opportunity to try out these dishes, either at home or in the classroom. We specifically tried to include relatively simple and everyday recipes and provide substitutes for possibly hard-to-find ingredients.

We would like to thank the people who shared their recipes with us, especially Mrs. Lim Lorna Hwang, Olette Trouve, Thomas DuBois, M. R. Ghanoonparvar, and Nawal Nasrallah. Thanks most of all to the project editor, Marjolijn Kaiser, who assembled the material, supervised the editing, located new authors and happily tested out the recommended (vegetarian) recipes.

East Asia

Chinese Cuisine

Known for their variety and inventiveness, the regional cuisines of China are enjoyed across the world and have evolved over a history stretching for thousands of years. Although covering vastly different landscapes and geographies, China has for much of its history been a land of scarcity, where the mostly agricultural population learned to make use of limited resources. From the staples of rice in the south and wheat in the north, to the use of peppers in the southwestern provinces, to the love of soups and gentle flavorings in the southeast, Chinese cuisine is as vast and multifaceted as the country itself.

China's cuisine has spread to all corners of the earth, and the lavishness and variety of Chinese meals is legendary. Yet, through most of history, the vast majority of Chinese people have eaten very simple fare and have considered themselves lucky if they had enough of that. Dense population, unpredictable weather, poverty, and progressive environmental damage combined to give the country a reputation in literature as a land of famine. Only since about 1970 has China been free of major food shortages. The cuisine developed its sophistication partly through the constant need to use every possible resource with maximum efficiency.

History

Early humans populated East Asia approximately one million years ago. They lived by hunting, fishing, and gathering plants and shellfish. Agriculture began before 8000 BCE in China. Recent finds have shown that by this time, rice agriculture was well established along the Yangtze (Chang) River and agriculture based on foxtail millet *(Setaria italica)* was established in the drier, cooler drainage basin of the Yellow River (Huanghe). By 4000 BCE, the cultivation or domestication of many of the basic elements of Chinese food was already widespread: rice, Chinese cabbage, pigs, chickens, sheep, cattle, and various fruits and nuts. Hunting and fishing were still important, however. Archeological

3

finds have revealed that by 3000 BCE, a wealth of sophisticated cooking implements and eating utensils existed. Inequalities in wealth were also well established by this time. Perhaps wheat and barley had also arrived from the Near East. They had appeared by 2000 BCE, but were rare until later.

Chinese cuisine enters the written record in the Zhou dynasty (1045–256 BCE), when recipes began to appear in ritual texts. Supernatural beings and human elders had to have food prepared according to specific rules. The *Classic of Poetry* (*Shijing*), a collection of folk and popular songs from about 500–1000 BCE, includes the names of most of the commonly eaten plants and animals. Although the record of ritual cooking runs primarily to meat—always a luxury and feast food—and grain, with liberal amounts of *jiu* (mildly alcoholic drinks brewed from fermented grains, usually translated "wine," but technically beer or ale), the *Classic of Poetry* gives a wider perspective, with mentions of vegetables, fruits, nuts, herbs, fish, and game. Grain was the staple food, with vegetables a very long second in importance. The basic distinction between *fan* (cooked grain) and *cai* (vegetables, or any dish eaten with grain) was already being made. It continues to be basic in Chinese food. Soybeans were known, but not much used.

In the Han dynasty (206 BCE–220 CE), contacts with West and South Asia brought new products, including grapes and wine, and more importantly, advanced milling technology. This enabled the Chinese to do far more with wheat and soybeans, both of which need to be ground to be useful. It is probable that China's enormous wealth of wheat products—noodles, dumplings, breads, steamed buns, fermented pastes, sauces, gluten products, and more—began its evolution at this time. Soybeans were used for soy sauce and pastes, and probably for tofu (bean curd), though the evidence is thin.

In the next several centuries, Chinese cooking became more elaborate. In the Song dynasty (960–1267), growing prosperity and the arrival of new foodstuffs led to the development of the complex, sophisticated cuisine we know today. Crucial to this, according to modern scholars, was the development of a middle class. Unable to afford the sheer quantity of game and domestic meat that dominated the tables of the nobility, the middle class developed complex culinary techniques, making small amounts of ordinary ingredients into refined, elegant fare. Buddhism, which values simplicity, contributed to this development. In the northwest, Persian and Central Asian influences were particularly strong, due to trade along the Silk Road.

When the Mongols conquered China and founded the Yuan dynasty (1267–1368), influences from western Asia flowed into China, profoundly shaping court cuisine. Dishes from Baghdad and Kashmir were served along with Mongol and Chinese foods. Such influences remained primarily in the north and west. The east developed a highly complex cuisine that made much use of fish, shellfish, and vegetables.

The Ming dynasty (1368–1644), a native Chinese dynasty, reasserted Chinese traditions, partly because of a new nationalism. Cuisine perceived as central Asian became steadily less popular. Dairy products, for instance, were popular in west and north China during the entire period of Central Asian influence but lost ground during the Ming dynasty. Animal herding was displaced by grain agriculture in many areas as the population rose. Most East Asian adults cannot digest lactose (milk sugar) and get indigestion from fresh milk, but they once consumed much yoghurt and similar products in which the lactose is destroyed by fermentation.

The Ming dynasty saw the arrival of new foreign influences. Portuguese and Spanish traders introduced New World crops domesticated by Native American peoples. China's economy was radically transformed by maize, sweet potatoes, peanuts, tomatoes, chili peppers, tobacco, and minor crops from pineapples to guavas. Maize and sweet potatoes (and, later, white potatoes) became famine staples and animal feeds; peanuts were a new source of protein and oil.

The Qing dynasty (1644–1912), China's last imperial dynasty, saw a steady increase in European influence on China. The expansion of the tea trade integrated China into the expanding world trade in foodstuffs. After the fall of the Qing dynasty, the incorporation of China into the global economy proceeded apace. China has taken advantage of the global economy to spread Chinese cuisine worldwide. Such items as soy sauce and tea are now known and used throughout the world.

General Characteristics

Chinese cuisine shows similarities with other cuisines of East Asia, partly because of China's influence in the region. Throughout East Asia, meals are typically boiled grain with some form of mixed topping involving vegetables, spices, and soy products. Soup is abundant and important. The grain is most often rice, simply boiled (often miscalled "steamed"). Boiled rice (or a substitute such as millet or cracked maize) is topped with a mixed dish, usually involving a good deal of highly flavored sauce that can soak into the rice. Next most common, especially in China itself, are noodles—usually made of wheat, often of rice or other grains. These are most often cooked in soup, but they are frequently boiled and then fried with vegetables and flavorings (the familiar "chow mein"—more correctly *chao mian*—and its relatives). Steamed buns, small breads, dumplings, and other products—usually made of wheat but often of maize, buckwheat, or other grains—are common. These are usually eaten by themselves, as snacks or quick meals. In some of the poorest parts of China, heavy flat cakes of maize or buckwheat were staples. They have since been replaced by wheat and rice products over the last thirty years.

Within China, pork is the commonest meat. China is home to two-thirds of the world's domesticated pigs. Chickens—native to China—come second. Fish and shellfish abound wherever there is water. Thousands of species of marine life are used. Most fish are now supplied by pond farming. This practice was invented in China at least two thousand years ago and continues to increase. Hundreds of species of vegetables and fruits are eaten.

Traditionally, oils were most often made from cabbage seeds (rapeseed oil). Later came unrefined sesame, maize, and peanut oils, whose marked tastes added much to the cuisine. Today, rapeseed and soy oils are common; maize and peanut oils continue to flourish; all are refined and essentially tasteless.

Food is usually boiled, steamed, or fried. Soup is traditionally present at virtually every meal, and often is the entire meal. Water was (and still often is) highly polluted, and had to be boiled; making it into soup or tea thus made good sense. Frying usually involves the famous process called *chao* in Chinese and "stir-frying" in English: food is cut into small pieces and stirred in a small amount of extremely hot oil. This process spares oil and fuel. The custom of eating with chopsticks (*kuaizi*) was already established by the Zhou dynasty (1045–256 BCE).

The mix of spices and flavorings distinguishes Chinese food from other cuisines of East Asia. Flavorings in a Chinese meal almost always contain at least some of the following: soy sauce, fermented soybean paste (or whole beans), garlic, onions (often small green onions), chili peppers, fresh ginger, Chinese "wine," or Chinese vinegar. The latter two are made by the fermentation of grain, using special strains of fungi and bacteria that yield complex and distinctive flavors. In impoverished or climatically stressed areas, food flavorings may be little more than garlic and onions and a bit of soy sauce. In overseas restaurants that cater to non-Chinese, the flavorings are usually reduced.

Chinese cooking evolved as a cooking of scarcity. Several characteristics of the cuisine follow from this. First, food, especially meat, is cut into small pieces. This allows it to cook more quickly and go farther in serving, and makes it manageable with chopsticks. Second, dishes and stoves are designed to use little fuel. This, with the thin slicing, allows ordinary people to cook a meal on a handful of grass or splinters; until recently, this was all the fuel available for many or most families. Third, by putting small dishes of cut-up vegetables and meat on the rice, in a closed pot, cooks can produce a three- or four-course meal in one pot, cutting back still further on fuel use. These are only a few of the many tricks for saving fuel and food.

Another type of efficiency is gained by using almost everything edible. Tough leaves can be boiled for soup. Frogs, small shellfish, and minnows are consumed. Wild herbs and berries are sought out. Many crops are grown, the choice governed by what grows best in each local habitat—streamsides, rice paddy banks, groves, pots, even roofs. The result is an enormous variety of foodstuffs and of dishes. Restaurants often have four hundred dishes on their menus and can make many more on request.

Most important of all, Chinese cuisine is based on foods that produce an adequate diet on a minimum of land. Rice is the highest yielding of all grains. Sweet potatoes and other root crops extend the range of cultivation. Soybeans are high in protein that complements rice protein in the diet. Chinese cabbages and other popular vegetables are high in vitamins and minerals.

Many foods are eaten solely for their high nutrient value. An example is *gouqi (Lycium chinense),* commonly known as goji, or "the poor people's vitamin pill," whose leaves and berries are among the richest sources of vitamins known. Long before anyone analyzed vitamins, the leaves and dried fruits of this plant were known to be nutritious and strengthening. Handfuls of the fruit are used in soups for women recovering from childbirth or for persons convalescing from sickness.

Regional Variations

Within these general guidelines, Chinese cuisine varies greatly by region. The basic divide is between north and south. The north is dominated by wheat, with maize, sorghum, millets, and rice playing minor parts. The south is dominated by rice. The northern limit of the Jiang River basin is the approximate dividing line; the Jiang drainage basin grows both rice and wheat (and now a great deal of maize). Maize is produced in large amounts almost everywhere in China, but it is usually used for animal feed and is not popular with humans.

In the north, distinctive subtypes have evolved in the major geographic divisions. Particularly famous are the cuisines of Shaanxi (centered on Xi'an), Hebei (centered on Beijing and Tianjin), and Shandong. All are characterized by the dominance of noodles, dumplings, and steamed breads. All use a great deal of onions and garlic. Lamb, very rare southward, is used in the northwest. Shanxi food is simple and often flavored with local vinegar. Beijing food is more elaborate and has its own elite tradition in the form of the cuisine of the Forbidden City; the disappearance of the imperial court led to great reduction of this cuisine, but it survives in a few restaurants and banquet halls. Shandong food uses many vegetables, soybean products, seafood, and dumpling varieties.

The classic centers of the south are Hunan-Sichuan, the Yangtze delta, and Guangdong. Hunan and Sichuan have always had a spicy cuisine. Until chilies arrived from the Americas, the "heat" came from smartweed (*Polygonum* spp.), Sichuan "pepper" (actually a prickly ash or fagara, *Xanthoxylum* spp.), and black pepper and relatives (*Piper* spp.). Chilies gave local cooks a chance to escalate the heat level. This spicy style has spread to or has influenced most of southwest China.

Life in the Yangtze delta originally centered around several great cities: Hangzhou, Suzhou, Ningbo, Shanghai (recently), and others. Each city has its own variant of a general style characterized by sweet-sour dishes, much oil, a smooth and mellow texture, and very heavy use of vegetables and seafood.

Water Margin Pork
Shuihu Rou 水滸肉

Pork was the most commonly used meat in premodern China. Only recently have other meats, such as poultry and beef, become popular. In his classic 1974 cookbook *The Good Food of Szechwan: Down-to-Earth Chinese Cooking*, Robert A. Delfs write about this recipe and its origins: "The *Water Margin* (*Shuihu zhuan*) is one of the most famous traditional Chinese novels. Written during the Ming dynasty (1368–1644), it records the adventures of a band of errant heroes in northern China during the disordered times of the twelfth century. This spicy dish takes its name from the exotic fare of Mr. Jiang's wine shop described in the book's twenty-sixth chapter."

Ingredients
Marinade
2 teaspoons (5 g) cornstarch
4 teaspoons (20 ml) water
1 egg white (small)

Seasoning
1 cup (224 ml) pork or chicken stock
1 teaspoon salt
½ teaspoon sugar
½ teaspoon black pepper
2 teaspoons (10 ml) soy sauce
½ pound (224 g) lean pork, cut into strips 2 to 3 inches (5 to 7.5 cm) long and ½ to ¾ inch (1.3 to 2 cm) wide
⅔ cup (140 ml) cooking oil, plus more as needed
¼ pound (112 g) bean sprouts, washed, drained, and dark ends removed (if desired)
½ teaspoon salt
2 or 3 dried red peppers, seeds and ends removed
10 Sichuan peppercorns
2 to 4 cloves garlic, slivered

▶▶

Guangdong (Cantonese) cuisine is marked by its enormous variety of ingredients (even by Chinese standards) and its heavy use of various fermented soybean products, including the distinctive fermented "black beans" (Mandarin *doushi*, Cantonese *tausi*). Seafood is intensively used and often made into salty pastes and sauces; these resemble similar Southeast Asian products. Several other important southern styles exist, including Chaozhou (Teochiu, Chiuchow), Fuzhou, and others.

MINORITY CUISINES

Distinctive cuisines also characterize the many minority groups that speak non-Chinese languages. The largest of these, the Zhuang minority (speaking languages very close to Thai), is noted for heavy vegetable use and for certain fermented products. Some Zhuang villages are characterized by high life

---

Preparation

1. To make the marinade, mix the cornstarch with the water and beat in the egg white. Mix with the pork.

2. In a small bowl, mix the ingredients for the seasoning.

3. Moisten the pork strips with a few teaspoons of water and add to the marinade, stirring to coat.

4. Pour the oil into a wok or large sauté pan to reach a depth of 1 inch (2.5 cm) and set over high heat. When the oil is very hot, add the bean sprouts and salt. Stir-fry quickly until the bean sprouts are well heated. Transfer to a serving dish.

5. Heat an additional tablespoon (15 ml) of cooking oil over high heat. Add the dried red peppers, stir briefly, then add the Sichuan peppercorns. Stir once or twice, and then immediately reduce the heat and remove the cooked peppers and peppercorns with a slotted spoon. Let cool slightly. On a chopping board, cut the red peppers into slivers or small pieces. Crush the peppercorns with the side of a cleaver and then chop them a few times. Set both ingredients aside.

6. Reheat the oil remaining in the wok over high heat. When the oil is hot, add the seasoning (be careful—it will splatter a little) and cook briefly. Then, just before the liquid has boiled down, add the pork slices (drained of any excess marinade) and garlic. Reduce the heat slightly and stir-fry just until the pork has turned white and is done. Reduce the heat and remove the meat from the wok, arranging it on the bed of fried bean sprouts in the serving dish. Sprinkle the chopped red peppers and Sichuan peppercorns over the meat and pour the liquid remaining in the wok on top. If you like a juicier dish, heat an additional 2 to 4 tablespoons (30 to 60 ml) of cooking oil in the wok and pour it over the pork and beans sprouts. Serve hot.

expectancies, due in large part to their healthy diet of relatively unprocessed grains and varied local vegetables.

Tibetan food traditionally was based on roasted barley ground to flour (*tsamba*) and often beaten up in tea with yak butter. More elaborate foods, including pork, vegetables, and dumplings similar to *jiaozi*, have tended to replace this diet recently.

More distinctive, with links westward, is the cuisine of China's far west, the huge province of Xinjiang. Until recently, most of the population spoke Turkic languages and ate foods typical of central Asia and the Iranian world. Rice was often cooked as pilaf—stir-fried before boiling, purely a west Asian style (Chinese fried rice is boiled, dried, and *then* stir-fried). Bread is similar to Persian bread and is often a staple. Lamb or mutton is the major meat. Fruit, including apricots, melons, and grapes, is much more important than it is eastward; pilafs often include apricots or raisins. Spicing is sparse or may be influenced by west Asian cuisine (coriander, cumin, cinnamon); absent are the distinctive Chinese flavorings such as soy sauce, brown pepper, and Chinese "wine." Noodle dishes and dumplings, similar in appearance to Chinese counterparts, thus taste very different.

Current Changes

Chinese food continues to evolve and change. One change—deplored by traditional gourmets—is the overuse of monosodium glutamate, which was isolated from seaweed in Japan in the early twentieth century and only since the 1960s spread into Chinese cooking. Another addition is the "fortune cookie," invented by a Chinese bakery in California in the late nineteenth century; it reached East Asia in the mid-twentieth century. Western food, including the fast food offered at McDonald's, has come to China. Another recent development has been the spread of the Cantonese custom of making a leisurely breakfast of dim sum. The Cantonese phrase *dim sam* (Mandarin *dianxin*) literally means "dot the heart" but may more idiomatically be translated "hits the spot." Dim sum are small, savory, high-calorie snacks, most often various kinds of stuffed and steamed dumplings and buns. They are eaten with endless cups of tea. Traditionally a breakfast for workers or for weekend outings, dim sum has become exceedingly popular in urban China, and in many distant urban centers to which Chinese have migrated.

Issues for the Twenty-First Century

Today the Chinese diet is more varied and vitamin-rich but disturbingly high in fat, refined sugar, highly milled grain products, and—for many—alcohol. This trend has had a predictably negative effect on health; deficiency diseases have been replaced by diabetes and heart disease. Overuse of wild foods, especially rare animals (with the distinction between medicine and cuisine blurred), is now a serious problem. Erosion, deforestation, spread of cities and roads onto farmland, and other processes are destroying much of the landscape. Unless conservation is taken far more seriously, China may again be the land of famine.

E. N. ANDERSON

University of California, Riverside

Further Reading

Anderson, E. N. (1988). *The food of China.* New Haven, CT: Yale University Press.

Anderson, E. N. (2014). *Food and environment in Early and Medieval China.* Philadelphia: University of Pennsylvania Press.

Benn, J. (2015). *Tea in China: A religious and cultural history.* Honolulu: University of Hawai'i Press.

Cheung, S., and Tan, C.-B. (2007). *Food and Foodways in Asia: Resource, Tradition, and Cooking.* London: Routledge.

Coe, A. (2014). *Chop Suey: A cultural history of Chinese food in the United States.* New York: Oxford University Press.

He, B. (1991). *China on the edge.* San Francisco, CA: China Books and Periodicals.

Hollman, T. (2014). *Five flavors: a cultural history of Chinese cuisine.* Cambridge: Cambridge University Press.

Hu, S. (2005). *Food plants of China.* Hong Kong: Chinese University of Hong Kong.

Huang, H. T. (2000). *Science and civilisation in China: Vol. 6. Biology and biological technology. Part V. Fermentations and food science.* Cambridge, UK: Cambridge University Press.

Lin, H. J. (2015). *Slippery noodles: A Culinary History of China.* London: Prospect Books.

Mallory, W. (1926). *China, land of famine.* New York: American Geographic Society.

Mones, N. (2007). *The last Chinese chef.* Boston: Houghton Mifflin.

Newman, J. (2004). *Food culture in China.* Westport, CT: Greenwood.

Simoons, F. J. (1991) *Food in China.* Boca Raton, FL: CRC Press.

Tan, C.-B. (2011) *Chinese food and foodways in Southeast Asia and beyond.* Singapore: NUS Press.

Watson, J. L. (Ed.). (1997) *Golden arches East: McDonald's in East Asia.* Stanford, CA: Stanford University Press.

Traditional Chinese Medicine and Diet

Due to scarcity and famine across the millennia in China, farmers planted the most nutrient-rich grains and vegetables. Plants and herbs were used to cure ailments, and an entire medical system evolved around foods that were meant to keep the body's systems in balance. Many of these beliefs and practices are still common today despite the influx of less healthful products from the West.

T raditionally, Chinese food was very healthy, mainly because millennia of famine had led people to learn by trial and error how to eat to survive. But the Chinese diet has changed with modernization as more fats and sugars have become available. Traditional nutritional medicine worked well to remedy certain deficiencies despite being based on concepts very different from those accepted today.

Food has always been integral not only to the health but also to the culture of the Chinese people. China's traditional diet was adapted to scarcity. Before the mid-twentieth century, China suffered famine in some part of the country almost every year, and a major famine every two to four years. Malnutrition and starvation were the commonest causes of death. Enormous developments in food production took place but were counterbalanced by rising populations and by environmental decline from deforestation, cultivation of marginal lands, and similar processes that led to erosion and drought–flood cycles. The people adjusted by eating a diet that maximized the amount of nutrients produced per acre.

Most nutrients came from the humble, often despised everyday grains and greens. Grain staples provided the most calories and nutrients. Where possible, the more nutritious grains of wheat and millet dominated. Rice is less nutritious but yields far more crop per acre; it thus became the choice in places where it could grow well. Soybeans, another prevalent crop, yield high amounts of protein. Common vegetables such as Chinese cabbages, beans, and spinach are particularly rich in vitamins and minerals. The few animal protein sources—usually pork, chicken, and fish—were particularly economical to raise or catch and a rich source of protein and vitamins. Chinese women traditionally breastfed for a long time, sometimes three years, though usually half of that. Virtually all people in the past lost the ability to digest lactose (milk sugar) after early childhood. This, along with the lack of pastureland and ancient conflicts with herding peoples, explains the lack of dairy products in the Chinese diet. In the west, fermented dairy products are common. The lactose turns to lactic acid and is thus safely consumed.

Medical works from the Han dynasty (206 BCE–220 CE) show that the Chinese learned how certain foods corrected problems we now recognize as vitamin and mineral deficiencies. Watercress cured scurvy. Fresh foods and whole grains and beans cured beriberi. Red meats, especially iron-rich wild meats and liver, cured anemia. Goji (*Lycium chinense*) leaves and berries produced strength, vigor, and general health. We now know they are extremely rich in key vitamins and minerals and are, in fact, a vitamin-mineral supplement. They were, and are, used especially for women recovering from childbirth. Many spices have both mineral value and antiseptic action and were used to preserve food and improve its nutritional value. Diarrhea was effectively treated with broth in which fresh foods were cooked, an early oral rehydration therapy.

In the low-meat diets of ordinary people, lack of vitamin B12 was an especial problem. B12 occurs only in animal and fungal foods. The solution was soy sauce and other soy and grain products fermented by yeasts and fungi. The early Chinese, though ignorant of vitamin B12, found that such products complemented other foods and helped survival. Also important was bean curd (tofu). It provides not only protein but also vital calcium because it is usually coagulated with calcium salts.

Anyone with the means to survive could at least have a healthful diet. Studies by Cornell University in the 1980s and 1990s showed that Chinese living in traditional rural conditions had low levels of cholesterol (an average of 127 compared to above 200 in the contemporary United States), were lean and in good shape, and had low rates of heart disease, certain cancers, and circulatory and degenerative ailments. Some areas, however, showed high rates of cancer, possibly because of extremely low cholesterol levels.

The situation has changed in recent years. Meat, fat, and sugar have become more available. People prefer them to bean curd, vegetables, and unprocessed grain. The result has been a rapid increase in obesity, heart disease, and diabetes. Problems for the future also include specific deficiencies. Folic acid deficiency is an emergent danger because of the decline in vegetable and whole grain consumption. Folic acid deficiency is a major cause of birth defects around the world and may be increasing in China.

Traditional beliefs about food and health centered on ideas of yin (cool, dark, soft) and yang (warm, bright, assertive). Foods were categorized in various ways within this system. Early on, the ancient Greek system of humoral medicine reached China. It was known in the sixth and seventh centuries as still a rather exotic system. It fused with the yin-yang system and other Chinese nutritional knowledge. Foods were categorized as heating, cooling, wetting, or drying. Only heating and cooling remained important. In general, "heating foods" were high calorie and thus, literally, heating—calories are a measure of heat energy. "Heating foods" were generally prepared over high heat and frequently oily, spicy, or strong flavored. Examples are fatty meats, strong alcohol, fried and baked foods, and spicy foods. Some foods were regarded as "heating" only because they were of "hot" colors, red and orange. "Cooling foods" were low calorie, sour or astringent, cool colored, and bland: greens and other vegetable foods. Rice, noodles, and similar staples and moderate-calorie foods were balanced, at the midpoint between heating and cooling.

This system generally worked well because conditions such as scurvy and indigestion were considered hot and effectively treated with fresh vegetables. Anemia, tuberculosis, and general debility were cold and effectively treated with a diet of red meats, spices, and high-nutrient foods in general. Some "cooling foods" are also cleansing, helping the body to get rid of toxins or simply making one feel better by improving digestion and metabolism. The system did not always work, but it worked often enough to keep it as a valuable and functional means of health up to the present.

Another system was the consumption of "strengthening (bu) foods," considered to build body, blood, and vigor. These are easily digestible, mineral-rich protein foods, ranging from game meats and mushrooms to pine seeds and edible birds' nests (from the swift, Collocalia esculenta). These do indeed have nutritional value. Unfortunately for biodiversity, a less valuable belief arose that any strong, sexually potent, or strange-looking animal had special magical powers and could transfer them to those who eat them. Dozens of species of wildlife are now disappearing because of this belief, which, unlike so much of Chinese traditional nutrition, has been disproved by modern biomedicine. A less formal but widespread concept that does not stand up well is the folk idea that red liquids build blood, brain-shaped foods (like walnuts) build brain cells, and similar associations.

To this may be added the thousands of medicinal herbs and products recognized in Traditional Chinese Medicine. Many of these fail modern tests, but others are useful and have become worldwide remedies. The boundary between food and medicine has never existed in China. Foods are eaten for health, and herbal medicines are incorporated into gourmet dishes.

Chinese medicinal food has spread to the Western world through books, Chinese clinics, and medicinal-food restaurants. In China itself, restaurants serving *yaoshan*—"medical dining," or traditional medicinal dishes—have been growing in number and elaborateness since their beginning around 1980 in Sichuan. They serve updated recipes based on the medical-nutrition classics.

E. N. ANDERSON

University of California, Riverside

Further Reading

Anderson, E. N. (1988). *The food of China*. New Haven, CT: Yale University Press.

Anderson, E. N. (1990). Up against famine: Chinese diet in the early twentieth century. *Crossroads, 1*(1), 11–24.

Campbell, T. C., & Campbell II, T. M. (2005). *The China study*. Dallas, TX: Benbella Books.

Hu Shiu-ying. (2005). *Food plants of China*. Hong Kong: Chinese University of Hong Kong.

Mallory, W. (1926). *China, land of famine*. New York: American Geographic Society.

Mongolian Cuisine

Mongol foods reflect the heritage of a nomadic society. During the Mongol empire, chefs also developed a court cuisine that introduced new, largely Middle Eastern foods. Mongols also popularized distillation, not only of their own fermented milks but even, in the case of their Korean subjects, a hard rice wine, today's *soju*.

Traditional Mongolian foods were (and remain) whatever the Mongols could obtain from their flocks (above all, milk, usually consumed fermented; more rarely, meat, generally boiled) and by hunting or gathering (or today, by importing). They also fished. Today the Mongols also eat a number of bread foods when they can get access to flour or import them. These foods are often in forms borrowed from the larger Eurasian world, for example, the varieties of *boov* (from the Chinese *baozi*, meaning bread or bread food) that range from pastries to steamed dumplings similar to those eaten in China. Mongols also directly use grain, ground or semi-ground, in such dishes as *tsampa* (buttered grain). Tea is now ubiquitous, most popularly as *suutei tsay* (Mongolian tea), made by long boiling of compressed bricks of tea in milk, with various additives, including butter or cream, a drink almost always offered to visitors by yurt dwellers. Those living a more sedentary life have often assimilated the foods of neighboring Russians and Chinese. In Inner Mongolia, for example, urban Mongols often serve foods that are more North Chinese than Mongolian, strictly speaking, but these North Chinese foods themselves have been heavily assimilated from central Eurasia by centuries of contact.

Historical Record of Traditional Food

Hunting, gathering, and fishing, although disdained, are well documented in the fourteenth century epic chronicle, the *Secret History of the Mongols*, where no less a figure than Hö'elün-eke, "Mother Hö'elün," the mother of Temüjin, the later Chinggis (Genghis) Khan (r. 1206–1227), is said to have had her children

16

gather wild apples, bird cherries, various roots including garden burnet root and cinquefoil root, scarlet lily bulbs, wild garlic, wild onions, and garlic chives, as well as fish—small, "misshapen" *jebüge* fish and *qadara* (*Salmo thymallus*) fish—to survive. In general, such traditional Mongol foods, still eaten today in many parts of Mongolia, are monotonous, and access is highly seasonal and uneven.

International Taste

Mongolian cuisine was not always so dull as this description implies; the Mongols were once briefly arbiters of international taste, as is evidenced by the rich cuisine of the *Yinshan Zhengyao* (*Proper and Essential Things for the Emperor's Food and Drink*), a dietary manual presented to the Mongolian court in China by its author, the Sino-Uygur dietary physician Hu Sihui (1314–1330). In this work, whose recipes for traditional foods run the gamut from roast wolf to a Kashmiri curry eaten with what is apparently Indian rice, there is an underlying foundation of *shülen* (banquet soups). These are exquisite blends of lamb, spices, and ingredients from one end of Asia to the other, melded in an attempt to create a cuisine that has a little something for everyone but is, at the same time, firmly based in the Mongolian love of boiling.

In addition to such exotic combinations specially created for the court in China (and from it they spread as far afield as Mongol Iran and even Moghul India), the Mongols also served as conduits for the introduction of various exotic foods in more original forms, often as straight borrowings, but in many cases bearing the imprint of the cooking traditions of the time. One household encyclopedia (*Jujia biyong shilei quan ji* 居家必用事類全集庚) even has a collection of adapted "Muslim" (Huihui 回回) recipes. They combine Turkic influences (including considerable Turkic terminology) with mainstream Iranian influences, but the character of this mixed cuisine is clear, including a preference for mutton whenever meat is mentioned (Buell 1999, 219-222).

Beverages: Distilling and Fermenting

But all the food borrowings did not go just one way, as these examples imply. For their part, while they did not invent distillation and only applied existing technology, the Mongols greatly popularized it and created a nearly world taste for hard liquor, nearly all varieties of which are called *arkhi* or some form of the word, using the word that the Mongols adopted for their product from a local Arabic form. The word, in a Turkic form (*arajhi*), first occurs in the *Yinshan Zhengyao*, which also names at least two other kinds of distilled drinks, one with

Sweet Börek and Baklava

The following two recipes are typical of the household encyclopedia mentioned on page 17. The first is a recipe for a virtually universal Turkic food, the *börek* (a filled pastry made of phyllo dough), but the name is spelled in an older way. The second is the oldest recipe for what is unquestionably a baklava which may be a creation of Mongolian court cooks. The word seems to be Mongolian in derivation, although baklava is a Turkic form. The name *Güllach* is Turkic for "flower food."

1. [Turkic] *Chäkärli Piräk* [Sweet *Börek*]

Walnuts, 32 *liang* (Chinese ounces) (remove walnut skins using warm water). After cleaning and drying, pulverize in a mortar. Add 16 *liang* of cooked honey, 16 *liang* of roasted *kürshäk* [barley?] cakes crushed in the hand. Combine ingredients evenly and work into small patties. Use roasted *kürshäk* cakes to adjust consistencies of the patties. Use dough skins to cover the patties. Knead into [Persian] *sanbusak* shapes. Put into the oven and cook stuck on the walls of the oven until done.

2. *Güllach* [Baklava]

Evenly mix egg white, bean paste and cream to make a dough. Spread dough out and fry into thin pancakes. Use one layer of white powdered sugar, ground pine nuts, and ground walnuts for each layer of pancake. Make three to four layers like this. Over the top pour honey dissolved in ghee ["Muslim oil"]. Eat.

a Uygur name that is possibly derived from Tibetan. Among the new kinds of hard liquor appearing at the time, and at first called *arkhi*, was Korean *soju*, but this is made from rice and not the fermented milk preferred by their Mongol occupiers. According to the Chinese scholar Luo Feng (2012), the Mongols first became interested in distilled beverages because their favorite food, *airag* or kumiss, as it is known to the Turks—that is, fermented mare's milk—is seasonal and does not keep long. To maintain royal or princely prestige, some way of extending the kumiss supply had to be found, and this was the origin of distillation, since distilled kumiss, still called *arkhi* by the Mongols, keeps indefinitely. Although mare's milk was the preferred milk to be fermented for distillation purposes, the Mongols also ferment and distill cow and camel milk. This is one aspect of their food culture that has not changed.

The traditional stills used by the Mongols and, with variants, still in use (like the hard liquors made in them), spread far beyond the Mongol world. As the researcher Ana Valenzuela (2013) and her team have shown, the same kind of stills popularized by the Mongols to make their hard liquors are still used in Western Mexico, mostly by the indigenous population to make mescal, fermented from the agave cactus. This technology was brought by Manilla galleons,

Bal-po Soup

The following recipe is typical of the cuisine and incidentally the oldest known, pre-chili, recipe for a curry, with the heat coming from other spices. It shows the Tibetan connection of the *Yinshan Zhengyao* since Bal-po is the Tibetan name for Nepal and neighboring parts of Kashmir. It has a proper medical indication and then calls for the basic combination of large cardamom and mutton broth but also chick peas (peeled, as was standard in the Arabic world) and Chinese radish as basic additives. At least some of the mutton and the radish is to be cut up into small chunks, using a Turkic word to describe coin shapes. The spicing is mostly Middle Eastern, including *asafetida*, a typical marker of Iranian influence. Only the coriander leaves are probably from a Chinese source, although eating with vinegar is likely a Chinese touch too.

This recipe is not difficult to cook, but ethnic stores might have to be visited to obtain some of the ingredients, including the *tsaoko* cardamoms (Chinese food store, but any large, smoky-flavored cardamom will do), Chinese radish (Asian market), and *asafoetida* (Middle Eastern market). The other ingredients are not rare, but Chinese vinegar would be preferred for the vinegar, or a wine vinegar would work too. If you have a halal market in your community get the mutton there but any good quality mutton will do.

Ingredients
Mutton (leg; bone and cut up)
tsaoko [i.e., large] cardamoms (five)
chick peas (half a *sheng*升 [today about 255 ml]); pulverize and remove the skins
Chinese radish

Preparation
Boil the ingredients together to make a soup. Strain [broth. Cut up meat and Chinese radish and put aside]. Add to the soup [the mutton] cut into *sashuq* [coin]-sized pieces, [the] cooked Chinese radish cut up into *sashuq*-sized pieces, 1 *qian* 錢 [a tenth of a Chinese ounce or *liang*] of *za'faran* [saffron], 2 *qian* of turmeric, 2 *qian* of Black ["Iranian"] Pepper, half a *qian* of *kasni* [asafoetida], coriander leaves. Evenly adjust flavors with a little salt. Eat over cooked, aromatic, non-glutinous rice. Add a little vinegar.

Source: Yinshan Zhengyao 1, 27A-B.

which went all across the Pacific, from one end to the other, and their sailors, who often jumped ship and taught the locals useful things like distilling.

A Globalized Cuisine

Today, things are the same but also different. Many Mongols now live in the city, with fewer opportunities to raise their own livestock, although many other Mongols still raise sheep and goats. There are now more horses and camels, the former even eaten, a use for which they were once too valuable. World food trends affect Mongolia, too, like every other culture. Ulaanbaatar is awash with fast-food restaurants, from Kentucky Fried Chicken to MacDonald's, not to mention popular Korean restaurants. Russian influences are also pervasive in Mongolia, as are Chinese in Inner Mongolia. All of this has yielded some strange delights, like a classic soup, *shülen*, served with French fries as additives rather than the more traditional items such as chickpeas. But thanks to trade, for example with China, the public markets of Ulaanbaatar also show a profusion of foods imported from Turfan and other places outside what once was the typical Mongolian culinary experience.

Paul D. BUELL

University of North Georgia

Further Reading

Buell, Paul. D., & Anderson, E. N. (2010). *A soup for the Qan: Chinese dietary medicine of the Mongol era as seen in Hu Sihui's Yinshan zhengyao.* Leiden and Boston: E. J. Brill

Buell, Paul. D. (2006). Steppe foodways and history. *Asian Medicine, Tradition and Modernity*, 2.2 (2006), 171–2Buell, Paul. D. (1999). Mongolian Empire and Turkicization: The evidence of food and foodways. In Reuven Amitai-Preiss (Ed.), *The Mongol Empire and its legacy* (pp. 200–223). Leiden and Boston: E. J. Brill.

Buell, Paul. D. (1990). Pleasing the palate of the Qan: Changing foodways of the imperial Mongols. *Mongolian Studies*, 13, 57–81.

Buell, Paul. D., & Pablo Moya, M. (2016). Distilling of the Volga Kalmucks and Mongols: Two accounts from the 18th Century by Peter Pallas with some modern comparisons. *Crossroads* 13, 3 (2016), 1–9

Luo Feng. (2012). Liquor still and milk-wine distilling technology in the Mongol-Yuan period. In Luo Feng & Roger Covey (Eds.), *Chinese scholars on Inner Asia* (pp. 487–518). Bloomington: Indiana University Press.

Valenzuela, A.; Zapata, G.; Buell, P.D.; de la Paz Solano-Pérez, M. & Hyunhee, P. (2013). Huichol stills: A century of anthropology—technology transfer and innovation. *Crossroads*, 8, 157–191.

Japanese Cuisine

The cuisine of Japan is one of the most distinctive—and popular—in the world as a result of the island nation's history, which includes periods of isolation as well as periods of openness to foreign influence. Most of all, Japanese cuisine reflects the country's geography as an archipelago of islands with soil and landscapes suitable for growing rice.

The basic characteristics of Japanese foodways may be traced to their ecological and historical contexts, which include influences from Asian and European cuisines, periods of isolation from other nations, and above all, conditions related to island life. Reliance on the products of the sea made fish, shellfish, and sea vegetables preeminent in the Japanese diet, and the suitability of Japanese soil to rice farming made rice the staple carbohydrate. Rice is the center of any meal; in fact, most older Japanese would not consider a meal complete without it. Other dishes, such as pickles, cooked vegetables, and small amounts of salted fish and egg, are flavor accompaniments to the main dish of rice. Before modern transportation permitted a more varied diet, people ate whatever their local areas afforded.

Legendary Times Through the Nara Period

Prehistoric evidence from archaeological sites demonstrates the dominance of sea foods, especially shellfish—*asari* (short-necked clam), *hotategai* (scallop), and *awabi* (abalone)—as represented in ancient shell mounds. It is probable that fish such as *tai* (sea bream), *suzuki* (sea bass), *koi* (carp), and *unagi* (eel) were also central to the diet during the Jomon culture (10,000–300 BCE). In addition, deer, crane, duck, boar, and rabbit were eaten. There is evidence too of other foods, such as nuts and melons. Pottery and tools indicate that boiling and grilling were the main cooking methods. By the third century BCE, mainland Asian rice, millet, and wheat had come to Japan. Salt extraction from sea water permitted the pickling, preserving, and fermenting of foods; it was in this period

21

that the standard meal evolved, consisting of a central grain dish accompanied by small portions of pickles and vegetables.

Rice growing depends on the cooperation of many people and the coordination of irrigation systems. By the seventh century, reliance on rice cultivation helped to create a political and social system in which mutual dependency for labor and irrigation was managed and controlled by a landlord class that gained economic and political power. Taxation of agricultural production was managed by a bureaucracy that could reach every farm worker and tie local organizations and authorities to the imperial capital, which by the eighth century was established in Nara. The court at Nara received the bounty of the outlying regions, and a more diversified and elite cuisine became the object of courtier connoisseurship. Along with the refinement of taste, preparation methods were codified. Artisan tableware developed, and an aesthetics of dining manners was created for courtiers. Class distinctions in diet and manners were apparent. Chopsticks (*hashi*) were used by aristocrats, while common people ate with their fingers. Peasants, agricultural producers of the aristocratic rice, ate less refined grains such as millet (both fox millet, *awa*, and ordinary millet, *kibi*). Rice was sometimes mixed with a variety of other grains.

Heian and Kamakura Periods

During the Heian period (794–1185), court life featured elaborate presentations based on Chinese cooking methods. At the same time, the variety of foodstuffs declined under the influence of Chinese Buddhism, which prohibited the use of animal products. Japanese culinary historians look to this period as the time when the foundational and ubiquitous soup stock, *dashi*, was developed. Literature of the time includes details of dining including service and etiquette. While rice was clearly the staple food, noodles were also prepared. A banquet might include raw fish, a soup, boiled foods, grilled and fried foods, followed by more boiled and steamed foods, and ending with pickles and rice. Murasaki Shikibu, author of the Heian-period novel *The Tale of Genji*, records that the meals were taken at mid-morning and mid-afternoon, supplemented by snack foods during the day and evening.

In the Kamakura period (1185–1333), the dominance of the warrior class spread a culture of simplicity and tough frugality, in which it became a virtue to simplify one's meals. Indeed, going without a meal was seen as a sign of good character. A samurai might ostentatiously chew on a toothpick—originally the sign of a completed meal—but this for samurai came to signify the opposite, a sign of abstinence from eating. The need for foods transportable to battle sites and campgrounds may have been the origin of the *bento*, prepared foods that would keep longer. The *umeboshi* or pickled plum is said to have been created in this period; it became a necessary accompaniment to rice and other grains. In the court and in temples, however, refinements were based on Zen Buddhist simplicity rather than warrior sensibilities and on the tea ceremony, which was developed and practiced by Buddhist priests. The development of a Zen Buddhist cuisine elevated frugality and vegetarianism to an art in which "eating with the eyes" (*me de taberu*) was a value, and the aesthetics of food preparation and presentation became a tenet of Buddhist culinary practice.

The Tokugawa Period

The influences of European foodways began in Japan in the 1500s, when traders and missionaries from Spain, Portugal, and Holland brought methods of preparation such as breading and deep frying, as well as new foodstuffs such as leavened bread. Most of these *namban ryori* (southern barbarian cooking) foods, however, did not influence local diets beyond the more cosmopolitan samurai and official classes, as well as some social-climbing merchants. Moreover, there were as yet no routes to disseminate these novelties widely, and most people's diets were still determined by locally available foodstuffs.

By the Edo or Tokugawa period (1600/1603–1868), the elaborate cuisine attached to the tea ceremony (*cha kaiseki ryori*) defined an order of service and mode of eating. *Kaiseki* cuisine emerged as the most refined eating, and evolved as a formal meal independent of the tea ceremony from which it derived. Seasonal fresh foods were emphasized, and the quality of ingredients was highly regarded. *Kaiseki* service stipulated that each element in the meal be prepared separately to ensure freshness and that it be prepared according to its own nature. The idea of separate courses in a meal was established by this principle. As a correlate, the appearance of each dish became very important, and serving wares and implements were designed to reflect color and taste, as well as to present each element of the meal to its best advantage. A dish was chosen to enhance a particular food, and not to match other dishes in the meal. The order of service, as established and elaborated from the Heian period banquet, began with *sakizuke* (appetizers), tiny portions of elegantly prepared fish. Second was *chinmi*, a kind of salad, tofu, or wheat gluten. Third was a soup, often a simple and elegant clear broth with a tiny vegetable, fish, or clam decorating the bottom of a dark lacquer bowl, perhaps suggesting a miniature landscape. Next was *mukozuke*, a portion of sashimi or raw fish, followed by *takiawase* (a vegetarian simmered dish). There followed *mushimono*, steamed items flavored with a sauce based on soy sauce and garnished with grated *tororo imo* (mountain potato), a *yakimono* or grilled dish, a vinegar *sunomono* (salad), and finally rice with *miso* soup and pickle. Sushi in this era was often *funazushi* or *narezushi*, the earliest kinds of sushi (originally from Southeast Asia), in which fish was fermented for up to four years before eating with rice. Variations on these themes abound, and *kaiseki* came to include a wide variety of ingredients and preparations, combining the virtues of Buddhist simplicity with elaborate aesthetics.

During the Edo period, peace and bureaucratic centralization allowed for the flowering of arts and the development of an urban culture. The rise of the merchant class and a money economy meant the creation of a new urban consumer culture, which included an emphasis on entertainment and eating. Restaurants such as noodle shops, tempura shops, and grill houses became popular in the entertainment sections of cities. There were also *yatai*, stalls where workers could stop for a stand-up or sit-down meal. New foodstuffs continued to diversify the diet of the townspeople, and foreign ingredients and modes of preparation were introduced. Chinese traditions also continued to influence the diet in such foods as noodles and hot pot dishes, often arriving from China through Korea to Japan. The bureaucratic centralization of the nation included compulsory sojourns in Edo (present-day Tokyo) for local *daimyo* (feudal lords); the frequent travel this system demanded helped to establish regular routes to the capital along which restaurants and teahouses sprang up. As ever, social class distinctions were reflected in food consumption patterns. Elaborate entertainments focusing on food were popular among the aristocracy and some members of the merchant class. Among commoners and peasants, a much simpler diet prevailed.

Meiji and Taisho Periods

Western food traditions continued to influence Japan even in the *sakoku jidai* (closed country) of the Tokugawa period. It was in the Meiji period (1868–1912), however, that full exposure to the foodstuffs and cultures of the West occurred. At first many people were reluctant to try exotic substances, but the diffusion of a sophisticated cosmopolitan urban culture through media such as women's magazines—which included recipes for roast meats and dairy-based dishes like custards, puddings, and butter cakes—spread the fashion of eating foreign foods. Many older people, however, rejected meals based on bread, potatoes, and starches other than rice. Meat eating had arrived in Japan much earlier, when Spanish and Portuguese missionaries had made beef part of the Christian conversion experiences of nobles in the sixteenth century. Ordinary people, however, did not eat beef until the Meiji era. Some Meiji leaders encouraged the eating of beef as a means for strengthening Japanese physically. The Meiji Emperor proclaimed the suitability of beef for the Japanese diet, and dishes

Dashi and Miso Soup

In Japan, like in many other East Asian culinary traditions, soup is not served as its own course at the start of a meal but rather toward the end, and usually with a bowl of rice. In its most basic form, miso soup consists of just two ingredients: dashi (Japanese stock) and miso (soybean) paste. Dashi can be made using dried kelp (kombu), flaked and dried tuna-like fish (*katsuobushi*), or dried anchovies (*iriko*), or some combination of these. The process is similar for all versions: the dried ingredients are soaked in water, heated to the point of boiling, then removed from the stock. For miso soup, additional ingredients are added after the dashi and miso paste have been mixed, and although miso soup traditionally is simple and light, the combinations are endless. You can make larger amounts of dashi, refrigerate it, and use it throughout the week for various meals or multiple servings of miso soup.

Dashi
Ingredients
4 cups (960 ml) water
1 piece dried kombu (kelp) and/or 3 cups (36 g) dried bonito flakes and/or 1 cup dried anchovies
1-inch (2.5 cm) piece of peeled ginger (optional)

Preparation
Combine the water, kombu, and ginger in a large pot over medium heat. Make sure the mixture does not come to a boil, but once it is about to do so, turn off the heat and remove the kombu. Let cool and store in the refrigerator or use immediately.

Miso Soup
Serves 4

Ingredients
4 cups (960 ml) dashi
⅓ cup (90 g) miso paste

Preparation
1. Heat the dashi until steaming, but do not bring to a boil. Turn the heat to low.

2. In a small bowl, combine about ½ cup (120 ml) of the dashi and the miso paste, whisking until smooth. Pour the miso mixture back into the hot dashi.

3. Add any additional ingredients (e.g., tofu or mushrooms), but make sure that the soup does not boil; the miso will lose its flavor if it boils.

Source: Inspired by Mark Bittman's *How to cook everything vegetarian* (2007), and Namiko Chen's website Just One Cookbook (https://www.justonecookbook.com/how-to-make-dashi/).

like *sukiyaki* became popular. Western dining habits began to influence home meals. A dining table and chairs took the place of a traditional low *kotatsu* table and sitting on the floor. Using Western cutlery was also a novelty, and etiquette books became popular, describing the precise fork and spoon to use with a course or dish.

In the Taisho period (1912–1926), the Japanese began to create uniquely Japanese versions of adopted foodstuffs, as with the Japanese versions of British versions of Indian curries (*kare raisu*). Pork dishes like *tonkatsu*, using the Portuguese method of deep frying the meat and serving it with shredded cabbage salad, became ordinary urban restaurant food, as did *korokke* (croquettes), torpedo-shaped fried mixtures of potato, chicken, and other foods, derived from French and other European dishes.

Food technology also changed from the beginning of the Meiji period. Industrialization involved changes in household technology, as well as changes in agricultural and food processing technologies. Refrigeration in food locations, as well as in transport vehicles for fresh foods, meant a greater distribution of fresh foodstuffs and better preservation without salting, pickling, drying, and fermenting.

Globalization and Food Culture

Globalization produced new influences on the daily diet of most Japanese people. Fresh and frozen seafood and produce can be transported to Japan from anywhere in the world within twenty-four hours. In the early twenty-first century, Japan was the buyer of about 55 percent of the tuna caught in the world. The extraordinary period of economic boom demonstrated the full diversification and spread of the Japanese diet, as restaurants of high quality prospered and food trends became more elaborate. Eating as entertainment for clients, family, and friends became an expensive proposition, and meals of delicacies such as *fugu* (the poisonous blowfish requiring preparation by a licensed chef) could cost as much as US$300 per person.

The bursting of the bubble economy did not slow development of new food trends. In the 1990s, restaurant eating continued to be popular, although the business expense account for dining significantly diminished. Consumers continued to explore new cuisine, and ethnic restaurants became popular. (*Esunikku* food in Japan often refers to Southeast Asian, Latin American, and Middle Eastern foods, not usually European or American foods). Food-related television programs such as the hit show "Ryori no Tetsujin" (Iron Chef) became popular in the 1990s, along with food and cooking-related magazines. Food tourism also has become a prominent travel industry, with groups of connoisseurs visiting vineyards, restaurants, food-preparation establishments, and cooking schools all over the world.

Now that UNESCO has dubbed traditional Japanese food (*washoku* 和食) a World Heritage Cuisine, its global popularity has been "officially" recognized. Japanese food is known for its beauty, taste, and health, and has taken some interesting turns as it has traveled. For example, ramen noodles (originally from China) have been elevated from a common comfort food eaten late at night or after a drinking spree, to the inspiration for a chef's creative expression in America. In quite the opposite direction, sushi, a food not eaten regularly in Japan, but rather taken as a special and celebratory treat, is offered in western supermarkets in plastic containers as a take-away snack, and munched by college students in forms never seen in Japan—bristling with deep fried items, rolled in dragon shapes, or stuffed with cream cheese and smoked salmon. At the same time, in Japan, the proliferation of elaborate French patisserie, "authentic" Neapolitan pizza, and creative ice creams demonstrate the constant and vital transformations of Japanese foods at home. The UNESCO designation of *washoku* as epitomizing Japanese food might oversimplify the diet and ignore the changes in what is actually eaten by Japanese people.

Merry Isaacs WHITE

Boston University

Further Reading

Cwiertka, Katarzyna. (2006). *Modern Japanese cuisine: Food, power and national identity.* London: Reaktion Press.

Ekuan, K. (1999). *The aesthetics of the Japanese lunchbox.* Cambridge, MA: MIT Press.

Field, G. (1989). *The Japanese market culture.* Tokyo: Kodansha International.

Kumakura, I. (2000, February). Table manners then and now. *Japan Echo,* 58–62.

Kumakura, I. (2000, April). Tea and Japan's culinary revolution. *Japan Echo,* 39–43.

Rath, Eric. (2016). *Japan's cuisines: Food, place and identity.* London: Reaktion Press.

Seligman, L. (1994). The history of Japanese cuisine. *Japan Quarterly,* April–June, 165–179.

Shizuo Tsuji . (1980). *Japanese cooking: A simple art.* Tokyo: Kodansha International.

Tamura, S. & Kishi A. (1999, December). The impact of technology on the Japanese diet. *Japan Echo,* 51–56.

Korean Cuisine

Korean cuisine is renowned for its bold flavors, which include the ubiquitous kimchi pickle and fermented soybean condiments that are used as flavoring and relish. Barbecued meat, generally considered emblematic for Korea, is a modern invention, as meat consumption was restricted to the elites for centuries.

As was the case with other aspects of Korean culture, Korean cuisine developed under the strong influence of its powerful neighbor, China. Rice and fermented soybean products (soy sauce, soybean paste, and soybean curd or tofu) occupy a prominent place in the diet of the Korean people. The emphasis on five elements in Korean cuisine—for example, five flavors (salt, sweet, sour, hot, bitter) and five colors (red, green, yellow, white, black)—has its origins in the Chinese theory of the five elements (wood, fire, earth, metal, and water) and the importance of keeping these in harmony.

Rice and Meat

The technology of rice cultivation was brought to the northern parts of the Korean peninsula from China probably late in the second millennium BCE, but rice became a staple of the Korean diet only in the Silla period (668–935). Earlier staples had been buckwheat, millet, and barley. Before the late twentieth century, furthermore, rice was not the staple for everyone, but was rather a symbol of wealth. The old phrase "white rice with meat soup," for example, connotes the good life, while tacitly acknowledging that not everyone could afford either rice or meat.

Buddhist influences (according to their principles, some Buddhists should be vegetarians) did not have much impact on meat eating in Korea. Beef, pork, lamb, chicken, and various types of game were regularly consumed by the Korean upper classes. Still, before the economic growth of the 1970s, the eating of meat was a luxury for many people in Korea. Farmers, who formed the majority of the Korean population, rarely ate meat apart from the three days in

28

summer when dog stew was served and a special day in winter when sparrows, wild boar, or wild rabbit were prepared. In both cases, the eating of meat, which was not part of the daily fare, was intended to strengthen physical resistance against extreme weather conditions.

Over the last three decades, however, the concept of Korean barbecue has come to depict what is now generally considered to be a symbol of South Korean cuisine. Per capita meat consumption has doubled since the 1980s, and this shift could only be made possible by massive meat imports. By 2006, Korea was ranked globally as the sixth largest importer of pork and the seventh largest importer of beef.

Fermented and Pickled Products

The techniques of making wine and *chang* (a semiliquid predecessor of soy sauce and soybean paste) were also introduced from China and by the seventh century were already highly advanced. This was also the time when fermented seafood (*chotkal*) developed, along with vegetables preserved in salt. The latter eventually evolved into kimchi—the spicy pickled cabbage that is nowadays a symbol of Korea and Korean culture.

Kimchi is considered to be quintessentially Korean by Koreans and foreigners alike. Yet, in the form we know it today, it matured only a hundred years ago, after chili pepper and *chotkal* were added to the fermentation process. The addition of chili pepper took place in the mid-eighteenth century and gave kimchi its characteristic red color and pungent taste. *Chotkal*, which has been included in the pickling from the late nineteenth century onward, not only enriched the taste of kimchi, but also increased its regional diversity. While at the end of the seventeenth century, only eleven types of kimchi were classified, the regional varieties of *chotkal* (some regions use shellfish, others anchovies or other fish), which is now one of kimchi's vital ingredients, contributed to the development of several hundred varieties of kimchi. The vegetables that are pickled have also changed. Gourd melon and cucumber have been used since ancient times, followed by eggplant and Chinese radish. The Chinese cabbage that is most commonly used for making the popular *paech'u* kimchi was introduced only about a hundred years ago.

Chili pepper was brought to Korea at the end of the sixteenth century, most probably via Japan. It began to be widely cultivated a century later and by the twentieth century had become an integral part of Korean cuisine. In addition to being an indispensable component in kimchi, chili pepper contributes to the flavoring of the majority of Korean dishes through chili pepper powder and chili pepper paste (*koch'ujang*). Both are not only used extensively in the kitchen, but often appear as a relish at the table.

Eating Utensils and Eating Habits

A spoon and metal chopsticks are used while eating. Rice, soup, and other liquids are eaten with the former, side dishes generally with the latter. Soup and rice are served in individual bowls, but side dishes can often be shared by more than one diner. Nowadays, bowls are usually made of stoneware, steel, or plastic, but for special occasions white porcelain is used. In the past, the tableware of the upper classes changed depending on the season: brass bowls were used in the winter and white porcelain ones in the summer. It is considered inelegant to lift bowls from the table (contrary to the rest of East Asia, where it is customary to lift bowls up to the mouth).

The majority of eating-out facilities in Korea have two dining areas: one with Western-style tables and chairs and one with an elevated floor where customers, seated on cushions, dine at low tables. Similarly, most Korean households use Western-style tables with chairs on a daily basis (with the table usually in the kitchen) but share meals seated on cushions on the floor, at a low table with short legs, when guests are entertained. The most traditional dining device is a small table designed for one or two persons. In upper-class households, such tables were once laid in the kitchen and then carried to different parts of the house where family members dined, divided according to age, gender, and position.

The Typical Korean Meal

Throughout the ages, Korean cuisine developed two distinct types of cooking: home cooking of the common people, matured within the family and the province of the housewife, and the more refined cuisine of the royal court, with its intricate cooking methods and elegant presentation. With the economic and social modernization that took place during the twentieth century, the distinction between the two became increasingly blurred. The twentieth century was also the time of Westernization of Korean cuisine. This process was initiated during the Japanese occupation (1910–1945), when Western food and drink, such as bread, confectionery, and beer, became popular in Korean cities, and a Western-style food processing industry in Korea began. Some Japanese food items were also adopted into Korean cuisine at that time, such as *tosirak* (the assorted lunch box) and sushi rolled in sheets of seaweed, which was popular in Korea under the name of *kimbap*.

A contemporary Korean meal is structured around plain boiled rice, accompanied by soup (*kuk*) and side dishes (*panch'an*). The number of side dishes varies, from three at ordinary meals to as many as twelve at more elaborate occasions. Stews (*jjigae*) and greens (blanched or sautéed and then mixed with a dressing) constitute the majority of *panch'an*. A variety of seafood and a wide

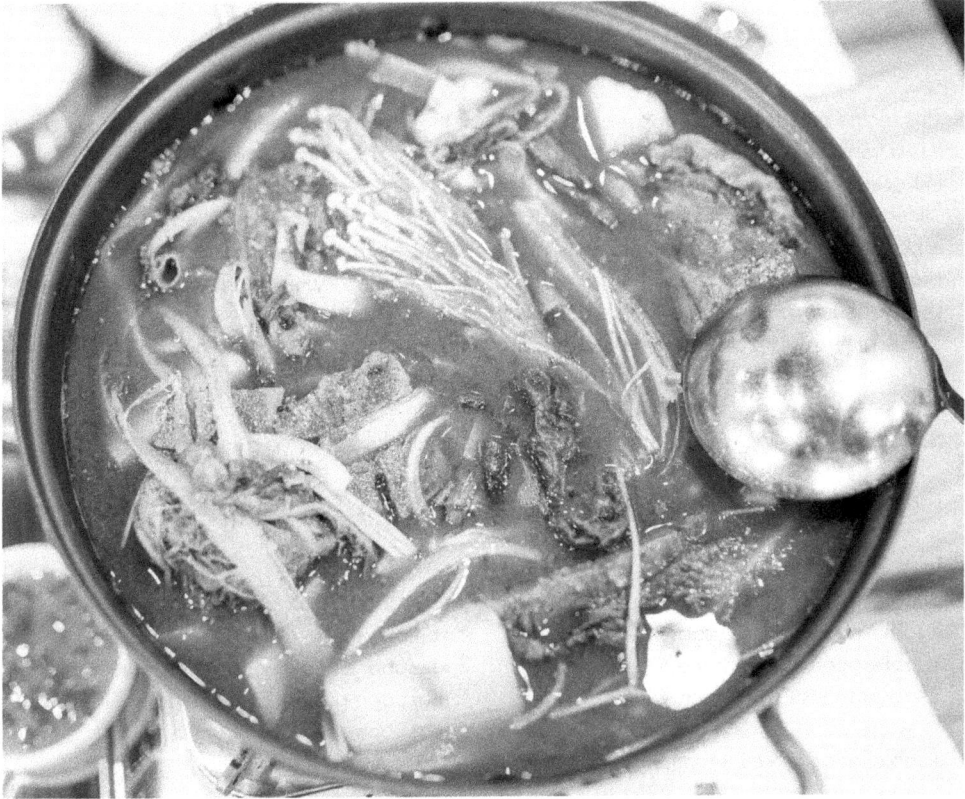

A Korean stew (*jjigae*).

selection of vegetables, along with beef, pork, and chicken, are the major food-stuffs. Seaweed is also used, but less extensively than in Japan. Chili pepper, soy sauce, soybean paste (*toenjang*), sesame oil, garlic, and green onions in various combinations give Korean dishes their characteristic flavor.

In recent decades, various noodles (*kuksu*) and stuffed dumplings (*mandu*) are popular and make for quick lunch dishes. Noodles are usually served in soupy liquids; stuffed dumplings are steamed, fried, or simmered in soups (*manduguk*).

Although the share of commercially prepared foods is rising, as opposed to the pattern of home cooking that prevailed before the 1970s, it may be surmised that further changes will take place in the decades to come. Change rather than stability characterizes Korean cuisine, as any other.

Katarzyna J. CWIERTKA
Leiden University

Grilled Beef (*Bulgogi*) Sauce

This recipe comes from a cookbook designed for those cooking Korean food outside Korea. It is a versatile, intensely flavored sauce fragrant with garlic and roasted sesame, so typical in Korean cuisine. It can be used as a marinade for chicken, pork, or (most traditional) beef. Sliced beef should be marinated for at least four hours before being grilled or cooked on a barbecue. You can use an inexpensive cut of beef, such as chuck, cut against the grain. Make sure you get a piece that is marbled with fat. The resulting grilled pieces of meat should be browned on the outside but still moist and tender inside.

    Sesame salt is a blend of toasted sesame seeds ground with salt, so you can simply use a little more sesame oil and some salt as a substitute.

Serve *bulgogi* wrapped in lettuce leaves, with kimchi and chili sauce, on a scoop of steamed rice.

For 1 pound of sliced meat

Ingredients

3 tablespoons (45 ml) soy sauce
2 tablespoons (25 g) sugar
1 tablespoon (15 ml) honey
2 tablespoons (30 ml) rice wine or dry white wine
1 tablespoon (15 ml) sesame oil

3 tablespoons (52 g) chopped green onions
2 teaspoons (9.5 g) chopped garlic
1 teaspoon ground black pepper
1 teaspoon sesame salt

Preparation

Mix all ingredients together and use to marinate meat.

Source: Inspired by Chang Sun-Young's *A Korean mother's cooking notes* (1997).

Further Reading

Bak, S. (1997). McDonald's in Seoul: Food choices, identity, and nationalism. In James L. Watson (Ed.), *Golden arches east: McDonald's in East Asia* (pp. 136–160). Stanford, CA: Stanford University Press.

Carter, D. R. (2003). *Food for thought: reflections on Korean cuisine and culture.* Seoul: Agricultural & Fishery Marketing Corp.

Cwiertka, Katarzyna J. (2012) *Cuisine, colonialism and Cold War: Food in twentieth-century Korea.* London: Reaktion Books.

Cwiertka, Katarzyna J. & Moriya A. (2008). Fermented soyfoods in South Korea: The industrialization of tradition. In C. Du Bois, C.B. Tan, & S. Mintz (Eds.), *The World of Soy* (pp. 161-181). Urbana: University of Illinois Press.

Kendall, L. (Ed.). (2011). *Consuming Korean tradition in early and late modernity: Commodification, tourism, and performance.* Honolulu: University of Hawai'i Press.

Kim, K. O. (2015). *Re-orienting cuisine: East Asian foodways in the twenty-first century.* New York: Berghahn Books.

Pettid, Michael J. (2008). *Korean cuisine: An illustrated history.* London: Reaktion Books.

Song, Y. J. (2006). *Korean cooking: Traditions, ingredients, tastes, techniques, recipes.* London: Aquamarine.

Southeast Asia

Indian and South Asian Cuisines

The cuisines of India and South Asia are among the most sophisticated, flavorful, and various in the world, with a multitude of influences that reflect the religions and cultures of the subcontinent. South Asia is a culinary and gastronomic hinge between East and West, evidenced in the cultural influences of the Mughal occupation and its courtly cuisine and the spice trade that brought new flavors from the Middle East, Europe, and Southeast Asia.

South Asia, most notably the modern-day countries of India, Bangladesh, Pakistan, and Sri Lanka, while incredibly diverse and composed of a multitude of cultural and religious influences, is unified in some ways by its cuisine. The most familiar and recognizable cuisine of the subcontinent may be Indian cuisine, but some of what passes for Indian food is actually Bangladeshi or Pakistani cuisine. The cuisine of each locality and ethnic group in the subcontinent was usually inspired by local ingredients, and each region boasts distinct specialties and recipes handed down from generation to generation.

Culinary Regions

Some of the distinctive culinary regions of South Asia are the Punjab area in the central Indo-Gangetic plain, including parts of Pakistan, dominated by spicy baked meats (such as tandoori chicken) and flatbreads made of wheat flour; the Bengal region to the east, including Bangladesh, known for mustard-spiced fish dishes and *rosogollas* (cottage-cheese sweets); the Tamil/Kerala area in the south, including Sri Lanka, known for rice-based meals, snacks such as *idli* (steamed rice cakes), and meat and vegetables cooked in rich coconut sauces (*sambol* or *sambhal*); and the Kashmiri region in the Himalayas, influenced by Afghan cuisine, with meat and rice cooked Persian-fashion with raisins and nuts.

The use of spices and sauces is the unifying thread of an otherwise diverse cuisine, as is the variety of unleavened flatbreads made with wheat flour, rice, and ground legumes. Dairy products, such as ghee (clarified butter), buttermilk, and curds (yoghurt), along with dals (dried peas and beans) and vegetables, are dietary staples. Vegetables are generally fried to make curry (or *kari* in Tamil) or are served with gravies or in legume-based soups.

A traditional meal (*thali*) for lunch or dinner is eaten with the fingers. Originally served on a leaf, now commonly served on a stainless-steel platter, a typical meal includes several vegetable dishes, rice, *puris* or chapatis (fried unleavened bread), pickles, *papads* (lentil wafers), salads, dessert, and yoghurt. The *thali* can be vegetarian or can include meat dishes. The meal is usually accompanied by tea, coffee, or hot water and followed by a *paan* (betel leaf and nut, eaten as a digestive).

South Asian cuisine also offers much in the way of vegetarian and nonvegetarian snack foods. These are usually savory dishes served with chutneys and pickles and eaten at any time of day.

Cooking in the subcontinent was traditionally associated with religious practices and moral beliefs. For example, India has a centuries-old tradition of cooking highly sophisticated and elaborate ritual food (*prasadam*) for sacred offerings to temple deities and for life-cycle rituals of devotees. This tradition is still alive today, and there is a vast resource of indigenous cooking knowledge and expertise in the subcontinent.

Diets and dietary restrictions in the subcontinent are closely linked to religion. India is predominantly Hindu, and while it is sometimes mistakenly believed that all Hindus are vegetarian, the practice is usually confined to the Hindu upper castes; lower castes eat meat such as poultry and mutton, but no beef. Muslims of India, Pakistan, and Bangladesh eat mutton, beef, poultry, and seafood, but no pork. Christians of the subcontinent eat poultry, fish, pork, mutton, and beef on a regular basis.

Vegetarianism

Toward the end of the Vedic period (1500–500 BCE), the concept of vegetarianism arose in the subcontinent primarily as a reaction to the dissolute upper castes who ate meat and drank liquor. The Buddhist notion of *ahimsa* (nonviolence) forbade the killing of animals as food, and this idea further influenced the Hindus not to eat meat. Asoka (d. 238 or 232 BCE), the Buddhist ruler of three-fourths of the subcontinent, further contributed to the development of vegetarianism by banning meat eating in his empire. Upper castes adopted vegetarianism soon afterward, and today vegetarianism is linked with upper-caste diet and behavior. Lower castes adopted vegetarianism as part of the process of Sanskritization (emulation of higher castes). Many vegetarian dishes

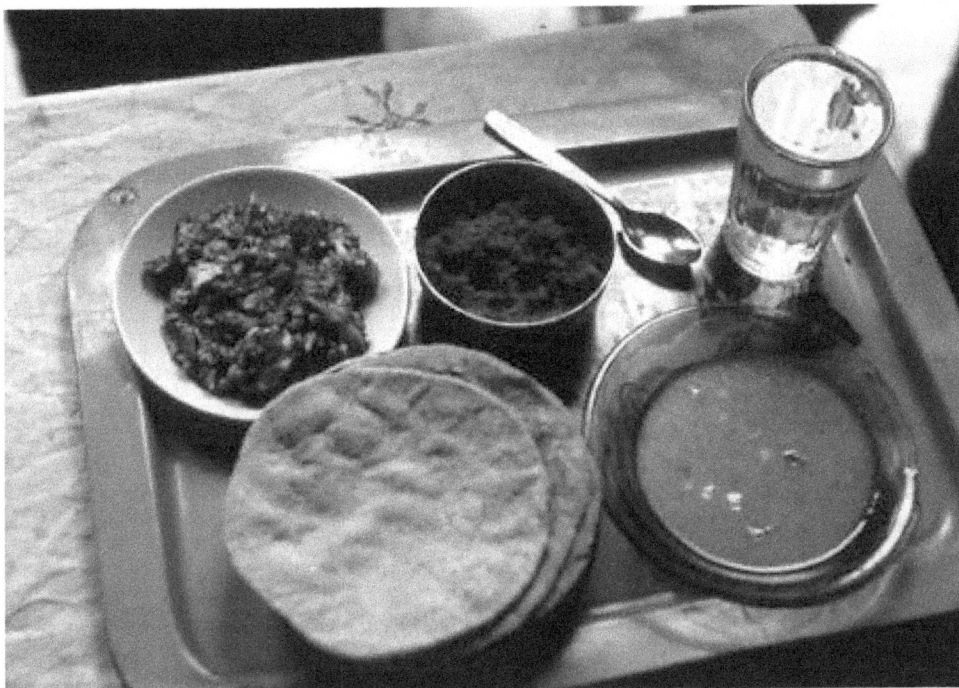

A typical homemade meal from South Asia, including roti, scrambled eggs, and chickpea dal.

of contemporary South Asia, especially of India, have been exported to the West, especially for those cultivating a healthful alternative lifestyle.

Historical Influences

From the second through fourteenth centuries, traders were constantly arriving in ports in South Asia on the spice trade routes that connected Southeast Asia, the Middle East, and Europe. These foreign elements inevitably seeped into the culinary culture and modified the local cuisines of these port cities and then the entire continent. The major influences from the fourteenth century onwards were the Mughals, the Portuguese, and the British.

In 1527, the Mongol emperor Zahir-ud-Din Muhammad (Babur) invaded India and established the Mughal dynasty (1526–1857). The Mughals created the "Mughlai" court cuisine, heavily influenced by Afghan and Central Asian cuisine. Spices were added to cream and butter, rice was cooked with meat, and dishes were garnished with nuts. India was also introduced to kebabs and pilafs during this time, as well as a variety of sweets made of wheat, cream, honey, and nuts. Today Mughlai cuisine forms the core of the cuisines of India, Pakistan, and Bangladesh.

Spinach Greens

Palak Saag

Spinach greens, or *palak saag*, is a traditional winter dish from the Punjab region in northern India and Pakistan. It can be made using various leafy greens, including spinach, mustard leaf, or radish greens. This recipe uses just spinach, since it is easiest to get in most countries. This dish is often served with a corn flatbread, called *makki di roti*.

Ingredients
2½ cups (500 g) loosely packed spinach leaves, washed and chopped
2 large onions, chopped
2 or 3 medium tomatoes, chopped
One 1-inch (2.5 cm) piece of ginger, peeled and chopped
4 or 5 cloves garlic, chopped
2 green chilies, chopped (plus more for garnish, optional)
1 teaspoon salt
1 tablespoon (8 g) cornstarch
2 to 3 tablespoons (30–40 g) ghee, clarified butter, or oil, plus more (optional) for serving
1 teaspoon ground coriander
1 teaspoon chili powder
½ teaspoon garam masala

Preparation

1. To make the *saag*, combine the spinach, half the onion, tomatoes, ginger, garlic, green chili, and salt in a large pot. Add about 1 to 1½ cups (240 to 260 ml) of water to the pot and bring to a boil. Cook for 7 to 10 minutes, until the vegetables start to become soft and the spinach wilts.

2. Cool the mixture and transfer it to a blender or food processor, or use an immersion blender. Add the cornstarch and blend the ingredients into a smooth paste.

3. Return the spinach *saag* to the pot and simmer for another 10 minutes or so, until it starts to thicken.

4. In a large skillet, heat the ghee over medium heat and fry the remaining onion until it starts to get brown.

5. Add the spinach *saag* to the skillet, together with the ground coriander, chili powder, and garam masala, and simmer once more for 3 to 4 minutes.

6. To serve, top the spinach *saag* with some ghee and additional chopped chilies, if desired. Serve with flatbread (roti) or rice.

Source: Inspired by Dassana Amit's website Veg Recipes of India (http://www.vegrecipesofindia.com/palak-saag-punjabi-palak-saag/).

The Portuguese travelled to Goa on the southwestern coast of India to trade as early as 1510, and Portuguese rule in Goa lasted for 450 years. Portuguese traders introduced New World crops to Goa, such as potatoes, tomatoes, chilies, pineapples, yams, tobacco, and guavas, transforming the cuisine of the entire subcontinent.

In 1600, the British East India Company was established under a royal charter of Queen Elizabeth I for a fifteen-year period of spice trading. That event marked the beginning of the British Empire's rule, which lasted three centuries on the subcontinent. With the British came a new cuisine called Raj—a compromise between British cuisine and that of the subcontinent. Bombay duck (native dried fish) replaced kippers at the colonial British breakfast table, and Bengali breakfast foods such as *kedgeree* (steamed rice and pulses) were exported from the subcontinent to the British table.

The British also introduced the word "curry," which people today associate with food from the subcontinent. British cooks ground spice powders to season meats and vegetables and cooked them into a *kari*, a stir-fried preparation with gravy. The British called the ground spices "curry powder" and took it back to Britain, where it became popular. In 1997, Britain declared curry Britain's national dish, and in a countrywide survey 51 percent of people claimed they were "curryaholics," a word that may soon be listed in the Oxford English dictionary.

South Asian Foodstuffs Abroad

In the indigenous food industry, Indian, Pakistani, Bengali, and other regional recipes have been simplified over time, and a wide range of prepared foods such as snacks, spice powders, lentil wafers, pickles, and chutneys are also exported for consumption by the South Asian diaspora and others who have come to love these cuisines by way of their travels, reading, or local Indian or Pakistani restaurants. Whether it is chai tea, *chana masala* (chickpea stew), or a simplified butter chicken recipe that one can make at home, the cuisines and foodstuffs of South Asia have become a global phenomenon.

Tulasi SRINIVAS

Emerson College

Further Reading

Achaya, K. T. (2014). *A historical dictionary of Indian food.* Oxford, UK: Oxford University Press.

Appadurai, A. (1988). How to make a national cuisine: Cookbooks in contemporary India. *Society for the Comparative Study of Society and History,* 4175/88/1193-0110: 2–23.

Ashokan, Anil. (2008). *Contemporary Indian cuisine.* London: Apple.

Banerji, Chitrita. (2007). *Land of milk and honey: Travels in the history of Indian food.* Oxford, UK: Seagull Books.

Burton, David. (1993). *The Raj at table: A culinary history of the British in India.* London: Faber and Faber.

Dassanayaka, Channa, & Ward, Natalee. (2003). *Sri Lankan flavours: A journey through the island's food and culture.* South Yarra, Australia: Hardie Grant Books.

Davidson, Alan, & Jaine, Tom. (2014). *Moghul cuisine.* Oxford, UK: Oxford University Press.

Frost, Cara. (2009). *Indian food & folklore.* London: Bounty Books.

Makan, Chetna. (2017). *Chai, chaat & chutney: A street food journey through India.* London: Mitchell Beazley Publishers.

Manfield, Christine, & Smart, Anson. (2011). *Tasting India.* London: Conran Octopus.

Marriott, M. (1968). Caste ranking and food transactions: A matrix analysis. In M. Singer and B. S. Cohn (Eds.), *Structure and change in Indian society.* Chicago, IL: Aldine.

O'Brien, Charmaine. (2013). *The Penguin food guide to India.* London: Penguin Random House.

Ray, Krishnendu, & Srinivas, Tulasi. (2012). *Curried cultures: globalization, food, and South Asia.* Berkeley: University of California Press.

Ray, Utsa. (2015). *Culinary culture in colonial India: a cosmopolitan platter and the middle-class.* New Delhi: Cambride University Press.

Sen, Colleen Taylor. (2009). *Curry: a global history.* London: Reaktion Books.

Sen, Colleen Taylor. (2015). *Feasts and fasts: a history of food in India.* London: Reaktion Books.

Srinivas, Tulasi. (2002) A tryst with destiny: Cultural globalization in India. In P. L. Berger and S. P. Huntington (Eds.), *Many globalizations.* New York: Oxford University Press.

Thieme, John, & Raja, Ira. (2009). *The table is laid: The Oxford anthology of South Asian food writing.* New Delhi: Oxford India Paperbacks.

Thai Cuisine

Food has been an integral part of Thai culture for centuries, and Thai cuisine is known worldwide for being both flavorful and spicy. It is distinctive among the cuisines of Southeast Asia for its great variety, its adaptive borrowing from other cuisines, and its global popularity. Thai cuisine is also diverse, with products and flavors that vary among its geographic regions.

"In the water there are fish and in the fields there is rice."
Famous Siamese proverb

"Food is a major cultural marker."
Jon R. Wendt

A common greeting in Thailand is, "Have you eaten rice yet?" Yet this only begins to show the importance of food as an integral part of Thai culture. Recognized globally for its diverse, spicy, and tangy flavors, Thai food reflects Thai culture as well as its geography, climate, and outside influences.

Food is also an important part of the Thai economy. For decades, Thailand has been one of the world's top rice exporters, and it is now also a major exporter of other food products such as shrimp and processed fruits. One of Thailand's major corporate conglomerates is Charoen Phokphand (CP), which started as a small local Chinese agricultural seed company. It now does extensive contract farming for foods such as chicken and manages the huge network of 7-Eleven stores pervasive throughout the urban areas of Thailand. Thailand, like Argentina, is normally one of the countries importing the least amount of food per year.

The Distinctive Nature of Thai Food

Thai cuisine is distinctive in several ways. First, Thai food is incredibly varied, with many different kinds of rice, fruits, vegetables, fish, and meat. As an example, there are approximately fourteen thousand varieties of rice that have been cultivated in Thailand, each with an economic and social role (Lofgren 2001).

Second, many Thais in rural areas live in a way that has been called *affluent subsistence*. Though they may be poor economically, they have a healthy diet comprised primarily of fish, rice, and fresh vegetables and fruit.

Third, other Asian and Western countries have influenced Thai cuisine, but the Thai are adept at *adapting* foods from other countries and cultures. They will take dishes like satay (from Indonesia and Malaysia), Hainan white chicken (*kao man kai*) from China, rice congee soup (*jok*) also from China, Kobe steak from Japan, and wiener schnitzel from Austria and adapt them to local tastes, which usually means making them even more flavorful and spicy.

Fourth, Thai cuisine has spread across the globe, and Thailand has been referred to as the "kitchen of the world." There are now Thai restaurants in nearly every country of the world, and exported Thai foods are common in food markets across the globe, particularly Asian groceries. Many consumers in the United States and Japan purchase Thai shrimp at their local food shops. There are about four hundred Thai restaurants in the Sydney area alone, and there is even a directory of Thai restaurants in Africa (NCC 2000).

The most famous Thai food product is the energy drink Red Bull (*kating daeng*) which has become extremely popular across the globe. In Thailand, Red Bull is actually marketed and labeled as a pharmaceutical product and contains high levels of caffeine and honey to foster alertness and energy.

The Character of Thai Cuisine

A typical Thai meal consists of several dishes, including a soup, a curry, a fried dish, and a spicy salad accompanied by rice. Food is normally shared. A fork and spoon are the usual Thai eating utensils; chopsticks may be used for noodles and in Chinese restaurants. Fresh fruit to cleanse the palate typically follows the meal. Thai cuisine is defined by its balance of four flavors: spicy, salty, sweet, and sour. Thai food is one of the spiciest world cuisines, and the world's spiciest chilies are grown in Thailand (Floyd 2006). Preserved fish, seafood, and fish sauce (*nam pla*) generally provide the salty flavor, while the spiciness originates from red chilies and peppercorns. Palm sugar and coconut milk lend sweetness, and sour or citrus flavors come from lemongrass, kaffir lime, and tamarind. Indian, Chinese, and Western cooking have influenced Thai cuisine, which also shares similarities with the cuisine of Thailand's neighboring countries: Malaysia, Myanmar (Burma), Laos, Cambodia, and Vietnam.

The foundation of Thai food is rice. Jasmine rice is the staple in central Thailand, while most people living in the north and northeast prefer a glutinous or sticky rice. Many of the diverse Thai noodle dishes were adapted from the Chinese. Abundant rivers, canals, and coastal areas make fish and seafood, either fresh or in a preserved form such as fish sauce, shrimp paste, or fermented fish, another staple of Thai diets. Signature Thai dishes are *tom yang kung* (lemongrass shrimp soup) and *pad thai* (a tasty dried noodle dish).

Fruit and Desserts

Located in the tropics with eternal summer and plenty of rainfall, Thailand has an abundance of diverse fruits. The province of Chantaburi is especially renowned as a source of high quality fruit, especially rambutans and durians (the king of fruits) known for tasting like heaven and smelling like hell. Other popular fruits include mangosteen (the queen of fruits, well-known for its health benefits recognized even by the Amish), mango, papaya, dragon fruit (also common in Vietnam), guava, pomelo, rose apple, lychee, sapodilla, coconut, snake fruit, and bananas—of which there are twenty varieties. Among the most popular of bananas is the short, thick *gluay nam wah*.

When it comes to desserts, sweets are generally eaten as snacks throughout the day or after meals as an alternative to fruit. Traditional Thai sweets include sweetened sticky rice with mango or durian and a custard called *sangkhaya* (made from Thai tapioca). Other popular desserts are crisp "red rubies" (made from water chestnuts), diverse custards, black sticky rice with taro (the rice is actually dark purple), coconut ice cream, and mango sorbet.

Food of the Four Regions

Thailand's four regions offer distinct variations of Thai cuisine, reflective of their climates, geography, and cultures. Each region has also been influenced by its neighbors, most notably the northeast by Laos and the four southern-most provinces by Malaysia.

THE CENTRAL REGION

Central Thai food, the regional cuisine most commonly found in Thai restaurants, is known for coconut-based curries and chili sauces and pastes. The food of central Thailand represents a creative amalgam of the foods of the four regions and is most diverse.

Central Thailand is also an area with many international influences, and in its urban areas it is easy to find various kinds of Chinese, Indian, Vietnamese, Japanese, Korean, Middle Eastern, and many Western foods. The Royal Dragon Restaurant in the Bangkok area was the largest in the world up until 2008, seating approximately five thousand guests with over five hundred waiters and waitresses serving food on roller skates. The menu had over a thousand Thai, Chinese, Japanese, and Western dishes.

With globalization now a pervasive influence in modern Thailand, particularly in Bangkok and the larger urban areas of Thailand, there is a proliferation

Pad Thai

Pad Thai, one of Thailand's signature dishes, is a noodle dish. Around the time of World War II, noodle dishes made by Chinese immigrants were wildly popular among Thai people, but in order to reign in the spread of Chinese culinary influence, Pad Thai was created using primarily Thai ingredients and flavors. It therefor contains none of the common noodle dishes ingredients (for example soy sauce or oyster sauce), and instead uses typical Thai flavors, such as lime, tamarind juice, and fish sauce.

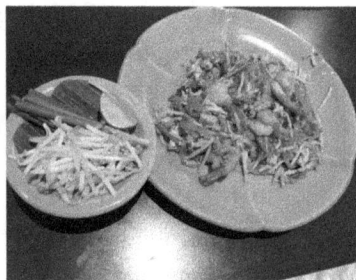

Serves 2 to 3

Ingredients
Sauce
3 tablespoons (3 g) palm sugar, finely chopped and packed
3 tablespoons (45 ml) water
1/4 cup (60 ml) tamarind juice
2 tablespoons (30 ml) fish sauce

4 ounces (112 g) dry rice noodles, medium size (2½ to 3 mm)
4 ounces (112 g) pressed tofu, cut into small pieces
¼ cup (38 g) sweet preserved daikon radish (*chai po waan*), finely chopped
3 cloves garlic, chopped
1 shallot, chopped
1 tablespoon dried shrimp, rinsed and finely chopped
½ to 1 teaspoon chili flakes, plus more for serving
2½ cups (250 g) bean sprouts, plus more for serving
1 cup (40 g) garlic chives, cut into 2-inch (5 cm) pieces, plus more for serving
¼ cup (35 g) roasted peanuts, chopped
2 eggs
2 to 3 tablespoons (30 to 45 ml) vegetable oil
8 to 12 shrimp, peeled and deveined
1 lime, cut into wedges, for serving

➤➤

of popular modern fast-food restaurants and shops such as McDonald's, Dunkin Donuts, Kentucky Fried Chicken, and 7-Eleven. This unfortunately has led to problems of growing obesity and diabetes.

Another fascinating aspect of Thailand's food landscape, and not only in the central region, is street food. With a huge informal economy, street food is most common in the urban areas of the country such as Bangkok. Currently, 11 percent of Bangkok residents never cook at home, and in certain compounds, kitchens are not included or allowed in the condos (for safety reasons). The most famous street food can be found in Bangkok at Sukhumvit Road Soi 38, where it is not uncommon to see BMWs and Mercedes Benzes parked along the road by street-food consumers. In the Sukhumvit Road area (Sois 4–23) all kinds of food are available around the clock, and on any day, even at 4 AM, there is

---

Preparation

1. Soak the noodles in room-temperature water for about 1 hour, until the noodles turn white and are pliable. Drain and set aside.

2. Meanwhile, to make the sauce, combine the palm sugar and water in a small sauce pan and heat over low heat until hot; stir to dissolve most of the sugar. Remove from heat, stir in the tamarind juice and the fish sauce. Set aside.

3. Combine the tofu, preserved radish, garlic, shallot, dried shrimp, and chili flakes to taste in a bowl. In another bowl, combine the bean sprouts, garlic chives, and half the peanuts. Crack the eggs into a small bowl.

4. Heat 2 tablespoons (30 ml) of the oil in a wok or large sauté pan over medium-high heat until hot. Add the shrimp and cook them, without moving, until they are halfway done. Flip the shrimp and cook on the other side. Remove and set aside.

5. To the same wok, add the tofu mixture. Cook, stirring constantly, until the garlic starts to turn golden brown, adding more oil if it seems dry.

6. Add the drained noodles and the sauce, stirring and tossing until the noodles have absorbed all the sauce.

7. When all the sauce has been absorbed, push the noodles to one side of the pan and add the eggs. Scramble the eggs gently and let them set about halfway. Put the noodles on top of the eggs and let the eggs set completely for another 15 seconds or so. Flip the eggs over using a spatula and break up the eggs.

8. Add the bean sprout mixture. Turn off the heat and toss just to mix.

9. Plate the noodles, top with the shrimp and the remaining peanuts. Serve with a piece of lime, extra bean sprouts, garlic chives, and chili flakes.

Source: Pailin Chongchitnant. (2016). *Hot Thai kitchen: Demystifying Thai Cuisine with authentic recipes to make at home.* Vancouver, Canada: Appetite, Penguin Random House.

much activity in this area. For the first time ever, there is now a *Michelin Guide Bangkok 2018* which dishes out accolades to seventeen of Bangkok's leading restaurants (Hsiao 2017). Regarding this new guide, the author states: "It changes Bangkok from the street food capital to the gourmet capital of the world."

THE NORTHEAST (ISAN) REGION

The people of northeast Thailand, Thailand's driest and poorest region, are known for eating sticky rice and *laap*, a salad dish made from minced raw or cooked meat, including that of water buffalo and catfish, flavored with garlic, chilies, lime juice, and mint.

The basic Isan diet is low in fat and it is characterized by spicy and salty food, with an abundance of diverse and tasty sauces. Other signature Isan dishes are papaya salad (*som tam*) and grilled chicken (*gai yang*). There is a famous cattle ranch of about 3,200 hectares, called Chokchai Farm, in Korat province, the gateway to Isan, which is the source of some of Thailand's best steak and quality dairy products. In the Northeast, exotic foods such as ant eggs and a variety of insects are sometimes eaten. Such wild foods are a good source of free protein (Prapimporn and Moreno-Black 2000). This region is slowly becoming more cosmopolitan, however, bringing in international and other cultural influences (Keyes 2014).

In the lower southern part of Isan, there are three provinces with large Khmer populations. In these areas, Khmer cuisine such as *amok* (*hor mok* in Thai), a wonderful seafood dish with red curries, is very popular. In Surin, organic rice is currently being promoted. In the northern part of Isan, in areas such as Nakhon Phanom and Sakhon Nakhon, there are many Vietnamese people, and thus dishes such as *pho*, a signature Vietnamese noodle soup, are prevalent.

THE NORTHERN REGION

Northern food is characterized by a wide variety of curries and chili sauces and pastes. Curries here are made typically without coconut milk. Pork is more popular in this region and frequently served as sausages. Given the adequate rainfall in this area, there is an abundance of locally grown vegetables and fruits. The signature dish in the Chiang Mai area of the north is *kao soi* (a spicy curry soup with flat egg noodles), which is unique to the region. This healthy cuisine has a low fat content. With the huge influx of guest workers from Myanmar to this region, more Myanmese dishes are available.

THE SOUTHERN REGION

Southern Thai cuisine, heavily influenced by Muslim Malay-Indian cooking, uses many spices, and the food of this region is Thailand's spiciest. The region is particularly known for its very spicy fish and other curries. Spicy, tangy salads are also a signature dish of the region. Surprisingly, though coconuts are prominent in the region, coconut spices are not commonly used. The majority of the deep south's population is Muslim and of Malay descent, so the influence from these countries comes naturally. Since many are engaged in fishing, seafood is a common dish in the south, with little meat eaten.

Signatures of Thai Food

There are three fundamental signatures of Thai food. First, it is a distinctive, highly flavored cuisine with an enormous variety of vegetables, fruits, herbs, and sauces. Second, it is a healthy cuisine, high in fresh fish, vegetables, fruits, spices, and herbs. A typical Thai meal provides a balance of proteins, carbohydrates, fats, and vitamins. Third, it reflects fundamental elements of Thai culture and tradition, including local wisdom which has been preserved over the centuries. An example of the Thai-ness of Thai cuisine is the aesthetic presentation of food, including the careful elegant carving of fruits and vegetables for special occasions.

Rosarin APAHUNG

Sang Nongthum School Cluster, Thailand

Gerald W. FRY

University of Minnesota

Further Reading

Alford, Jeffrey. (2015). *Chicken in the Mango Tree: Food and life in a Thai-Khmer village.* Madeira Park, BC: Douglas & McIntyre.

Counihan, Carol, & Penny Van Esterik (Eds.). *Food and culture: A reader* (2nd ed.). New York: Routledge.

Donnelly, Michael, & Nguyen, Luke. (2016). *Luke Nguyen's street food Asia.* DVD/video. Madman Entertainment

Floyd, Keith. (2006). *Floyd's Thai food.* London: HarperCollins.

Grimes, Lulu. (2008). *The food of Thailand: A journey for food lovers.* London: Bay Books.

Hsiao, Tina. (2017, December 6). First Michelin Guide recognizes Thailand's best restaurants. *CNN Travel.* Retrieved 4 January 2018, from http://www.cnn.com/travel/article/michelin-guide-bangkok-2017/index.html

Kelly, Matthew; Banwell, Cathy; Dixon, Jane; Sam-ang Seubsman; & Sleigh, Adrian. (2013). Thai food culture in transition: A mixed methods study on the role of food retailing. In C. Banwell; S. Ulijaszek, & J. Dixon (Eds.), *When culture impacts health: Global lessons for effective health research* (pp. 319–327). Amsterdam: Elsevier.

Keyes, Charles F. (2014). *Finding their voice: Northeastern villagers and the Thai State.* Chiang Mai: Silkworm Books.

Kummer, Patricia K. (2012). *The food of Thailand.* New York: Marshall Cavendish Benchmark.

Leela Punyaratabandhu. (2017). *Bangkok: Stories and recipes from the heart of Thailand.* California: Ten Speed Press.

Locricchio, Matthew. (2012). *The cooking of Thailand.* New York: Marshall Cavendish Benchmark.

Lofgren, Amy. (2001). *Thai rice: Trade, culture and freedom from GM seeds.* TED Case Studies, No. 635.

National Cultural Commission (NCC). (2000). *Directory of Thai restaurants: Africa, America, Asia, Europe, Oceania.* Bangkok: Office of the National Cultural Commission, Ministry of Education.

Nongkran Daks, & Greeley, Alexandra. (2015). *Nong's Thai kitchen: 84 classic and contemporary recipes that are healthy and delicious.* Tokyo: Tuttle Publishing.

Pailin Chongchitnant. (2016). *Hot Thai kitchen: Demystifying Thai cuisine with authentic recipes to make at home.* Vancouver: Penguin Random House.

Prapimporn Somnasang, & Moreno-Black, Geraldine. (2000). Knowing, gathering and eating: Knowledge and attitudes concerning wild food in an Isan village. *Ethnobiology, 20*(2), 197–216.

Stephen, Wendy (Ed.). (2008). *Thai cooking: Step-by-step.* Millers Point, NSW: Bay Books.

Temsiri Bunyasing. (Ed.). (1992). *Thai life: Thai cuisine* (4th Ed.). Bangkok: National Identity Board, Prime Minister's Office.

Thompson, David. (2009). *Thai street food.* London: Penguin.

Scripter, Sami, & Sheng Yang. (2009). *Cooking from the heart: The Hmong kitchen in America.* Minneapolis: University of Minnesota Press.

Vatcharin Bhumichitr. (1998). *Vatch's Thai cookbook: 150 recipes with guides to essential ingredients.* London: Pavilion Books.

VeLure Roholt, Christine. (2015). *Foods of Thailand.* Minneapolis, MN: Bellwether Media.

Yasmeen, Gisèle. (2008). Plastic-bag housewives and postmodern restaurants? Public and private in Bangkok's foodscape. *Urban Geography, 17*(6), 526–554.

Lao Cuisine

Influenced by neighboring countries and its own past, the cuisine of Laos is characterized by reliance on sticky rice, a wide variety of native plants and animals, and dishes flavored with ginger, galangal, and chilies. French colonization and more recent influences from tourism and the diaspora have shaped the cuisine found in the restaurants of large cities, while towns and villages retain traditional cooking methods and flavors.

L ocated in the heart of mainland Southeast Asia, Laos is surrounded by China, Burma, Vietnam, Cambodia, and Thailand. The valleys and plains of the Mekong River and its tributaries give way in the north and east to rugged mountains with steep limestone peaks. The cuisine of the ethnic Lao, the predominant ethnic group in Laos, is shaped by history, geography, local ingredients, and ethnic diversity.

Food and History

Present-day Laos traces its historic and cultural identity to the kingdom of Lan Xang (1353–1560), which was centered in Luang Prabang in northern Laos. Historically, the mighty Mekong River system provided water, food, and trade routes for the ethnic Lao, who developed food production based on paddy and swidden (dry) rice farming, animal husbandry, hunting, and gathering. France colonized Laos in 1893, uniting the Lao and other ethnic groups into the geographically bounded country of Laos. After several years of war against the French following WWII, Laos became an independent constitutional monarchy in 1953.

Less than a decade after achieving independence, Laos became embroiled in the Vietnam War. Victorious communists established a one-party state in 1975 and closed the borders of the Lao People's Democratic Republic (PDR) to most Westerners. The war and draconian communist attempts to collectivize agriculture produced many refugees. Those who stayed in Laos endured hunger or, at best, a diet of donated rice and forest vegetables. During the war, the United States flew more than 580,000 bombing missions over Laos—the equivalent of one raid every eight minutes for nine years. Today, unexploded ordnance makes significant areas of land unsafe for agricultural production (Redfern and Coates 2011; World Food Programme 2013). Thus, cultivating and cooking can be dangerous in Laos, which contributes to food insecurity, hunger, and malnutrition in rural areas.

Tastes and Flavors

In Laos, as in other Southeast Asian countries, rice is the daily staple; however, it is more than just that. Throughout the nation, rice agriculture, the primary farming activity, is an integral way of life. Ethnic Lao predominantly consume sticky or glutinous rice (*khao niaw, Oryza sativa*) that contains a large amount of amylopectin starch, which causes the kernels to disintegrate when boiled. Consequently, sticky rice is usually soaked, steamed, then served, or stored in a woven container. Sticky rice is so significant to the Lao that they consider it the essence of their identity and will often refer to themselves as *luk khao niaw*, "children or descendants of sticky rice." In addition to forming the main part of a meal, raw sticky rice is often toasted (*khao khoua*) to add a nut-like flavor to many dishes. Soaked and pounded into a paste, it is also used as a thickener (*khao beua*).

The Lao classify food in a variety of ways. Nicholas Enfield, professor of ethnolinguistics, found that Lao identify five main tastes: sweet, bitter, umami (the taste of glutamate), sour, and salty (Enfield 2011). Lao also use seven specific terms to encompass dimensions of taste, texture, and sensation: not salty enough/bland, hot/minty, biting/tingly, chalky/dry in the mouth, spicy/hot, causing an "itch" in the teeth, and oily-starchy-rich. Taste characteristics guide the combination of ingredients or dishes served with rice. These tastes come from local plants, resins, and roots primarily gathered wild from forests, ponds, and rice paddies. Consequently, flavoring imparts regional identification and a sense of tradition.

The qualities of taste, smell, and texture often accord with Lao traditional concepts of health. In this system, food is classified by the effect it can have for maintaining health or returning the body to a balanced state. *Hon* or "hot" foods heat the body, *yen* or "cold" plants produce a cooling and refreshing effect, while the third class is neutral and does not affect the body's balance.

Ingredients and Dishes

Lao dishes contain vegetables and herbs, rice or noodles, and small amounts of fish, chicken, pork, or beef. Vegetables, many wild, comprise the second most important food group after rice. Some common items are bamboo shoots, used in stews or boiled as a side dish; mushrooms, used in soups and stir-fries; *Phak lin may*, a bitter green, eaten raw; *Sesbania grandiflora* blossom, eaten as a vegetable in soups and curries; and *Phak bung* (*Ipomoea aquatica*), water spinach or water morning glory. Fruits, such as limes and bananas, are also important and often come from the forest or household gardens.

Food, cooked mainly by women and girls, served in small pieces fulfills the Buddhist custom that a whole animal should not be cooked and served. During a meal, each person takes rice from the basket, rolls it into a ball in their hand and then dips it into the communal dishes of food or sauce. Condiments, sauces, pastes, and fermented fish sauces add taste, texture, and color. These include *nam paa* (fermented raw fish sauce), *paa daek* (a thicker spread of fermented raw fish, rice husks and rice dust), *nam paa daek* (a sauce made from *paa daek*), *nam phak-kaat* (a paste made from fermented lettuce leaves), *cheo ngaa* (sesame paste), and *nam kathi* (coconut sauce) (Hays 2013).

Laap, often considered the national dish of Laos, is a salad made with raw or cooked meat or fish. Consuming raw food, especially fish, has deep cultural roots in Laos. Liver fluke infection from raw or insufficiently cooked fish, can lead to liver problems and even cancer of the bile duct. This is a major public health concern, since over two million Lao are infected with liver fluke (Phongluxa et al 2013). Grilling (*ping*) is a favored method of cooking; however, boiling, stewing, steaming, searing, and mixing (as in salads) also are traditional cooking methods. Stews are often green in color because of the large proportion of vegetables and *ya nang* leaves used. *Ya nang* leaves are soaked and squeezed to produce a viscous green liquid added to many dishes.

Religious Significance

Lao cuisine, and especially certain ingredients, plays an important role in Lao religious observances and events. Households support their local Theravada Buddhist temples daily by providing sticky rice and other food to monks and novices as they walk barefoot with begging bowls (*tak baat*) through an area. Providing food also occurs at temples as part of religious celebrations. The "animist" *baci* or *sou khouan* is a quintessentially Lao ritual and the central part of many celebrations, such as birth, marriage, ordination as a monk, traveling or returning, and the New Year. Food items are placed on the *baci* table. At a marriage ceremony, for example, bananas and eggs on the table represent the "many children" guests wish for the married couple.

Spirit beings are part of Lao beliefs. A spirit may inhabit a stream or a tree, or a guardian spirit may protect a household or a village. Food nourishes spirit beings, so household members may regularly feed their house spirit by putting a food offering in a miniature temple-like "house" designed for the house spirit. Traditionally, a village may feed its guardian spirit before planting begins to ensure the protection of their crops.

Modern Adaptations and Internationalization

While 10 percent of the population of Laos fled the country in the late 1970s and early 1980s, past Lao migrations had already affected and inspired the cuisine of the neighboring countries of Cambodia and northeastern Thailand. In 1991, the Lao PDR government adopted a constitution, and the country began to open economically and pursue regional and global integration. The internationalization of Lao cuisine grew out of the changing Lao economy and greater international familiarity with Lao cuisine through tourism and culinary entrepreneurship in Laos and abroad.

LAO CUISINE IN THE DIASPORA

First generation Lao-American households generally maintain Lao culinary traditions. They often reconfigure their American kitchen to accommodate pungent Lao dishes by adding a second refrigerator for storage, and a grill or stove in a covered garage or porch for cooking. Where there is a Buddhist temple, sharing quotidian and festival foods helps to create community (Clune 2016). Lao-American restaurants and small ethnic grocery stores help Lao families maintain food traditions while acquainting the general public with Lao food culture. Although many Lao-American entrepreneurs characterize their restaurants as "Thai," a better-known cuisine, the menus include Lao dishes, especially sticky rice and *laap*.

WESTERN AND TOURIST INFLUENCE ON LAO CUISINE

Western and Asian tourists are increasingly visiting Laos. Expatriate and local Lao are partnering with Europeans (especially French), Australians, and North Americans to establish restaurants in Laos. French influence on Lao cuisine is evident in the restaurant culture of Vientiane and Luang Prabang, the UNESCO World Heritage city, and in the French-style baguettes sold in town markets. High-end restaurants in the tourist core of Luang Prabang invite visitors to "enjoy a fusion of Lao and French cuisine" (Staiff & Bushell 2013, 133). Marrying Lao with French food suggests an exotic and enticing cuisine and is congruent with the patchwork of nearby French colonial buildings and Lao

Chicken *Laap*

Laap, often considered the national dish of Laos, is a salad usually served with raw or cooked meat or fish. This is a version with cooked chicken.

Serves 4

Ingredients
¼ cup (50 g) raw Thai glutinous rice
1 pound (450 g) skinless, boneless chicken breasts
Salt
2 teaspoons (10 ml) vegetable oil
¼ cup (25 g) minced green onions, white and green parts
¼ cup (10 g) fresh mint, finely chopped
3 tablespoons (7.5 g) fresh cilantro, coarsely chopped
3 tablespoons (45 ml) fresh lime juice
1 tablespoon (15 ml) fish sauce
1 or 2 small (1-inch/2.5 cm) fresh Asian chilies, such as bird or Thai, minced
Fresh mint, basil, and cilantro leaves, for serving
Tomato, coarsely chopped, for serving
English cucumber, coarsely chopped, for serving
2 cups (400 g) cooked Thai glutinous rice, for serving

Preparation
1. Roast the rice in a dry, heavy skillet over medium high heat, stirring constantly, until golden brown, 4 to 6 minutes (the rice will smoke). Grind to a coarse powder using an electric coffee, spice grinder, or mortar and pestle.

2. Thinly slice the chicken crosswise and cut the slices into thin strips. Season the chicken with salt. Heat the oil in a wok or heavy skillet over high heat until hot but not smoking, then stir-fry the chicken until cooked through, about 2 minutes. Remove the chicken from the wok and set aside. Stir 2 tablespoons of rice powder into the wok, reserving the remainder for another use. Add the remaining ingredients (except for the serving accompaniments) and stir well.

3. Mound the chicken on a platter and serve with a bowl of sticky rice and a plate of the herbs, tomato, and cucumber.

Source: Adapted from Eve Turow's recipe for NPR (https://www.npr.org/2011/10/18/141469615/chicken-laap).

temples. Tourist diners in Luang Prabang can experience Lao ingredients and cooking techniques in these "fusion" restaurants. "Chicken tartare cooked with fine herbs and spice," however, is in essence still chicken *laap* (menu item description, Staiff & Bushnell, 136). And in towns and villages, Lao households still prepare their customary cuisine, ensuring that traditional Lao cuisine will continue.

Geraldine **MORENO-BLACK**

University of Oregon

Carol **IRESON-DOOLITTLE**

Willamette University

Further Reading

Champanakone, Xaixana (2009). *Lao cooking and the essence of life.* Laos: Vincent-Fischer-Zernin.

Clune, Katy A. (2016). Home in a new place: Making Laos in Morganton, North Carolina. *Southern Culture, 22*(1), 95–112.

Enfield, Nicholas J. (2011). Taste in two tongues: A Southeast Asian study of semantic convergence. *The Senses and Society, 6*(1), 30–37.

Hays, Jeffrey. (2013). Lao cuisine. Factsanddetails.com. Retrieved November 13, 2016, from http://factsanddetails.com/southeast-asia/Laos/sub5_3b/entry-2958.html

Kislenko, Arne. (2009). *Culture and customs of Laos.* Westport, CT: Greenwood Press.

Lao cuisine. (2016). Wikipedia.com. Retrieved November 11, 2016, from https://en.wikipedia.org/wiki/Lao_cuisine

Phongluxa, Khampheng et al. (2013). Helminth infection in southern Laos: high prevalence and low awareness. *Parasites & Vectors, 6*(1), 1.

Redfern, Jerry & Coates, Karen J. (2011). The flavor of danger. *Gastronomica: The Journal of Critical Food Studies, 11*(4), 99–103.

Staiff, Russell & Bushell, Robyn. (2013). The rhetoric of Lao/French fusion: Beyond the representation of the Western tourist experience of cuisine in the world heritage city of Luang Prabang, Laos. *Journal of Heritage Tourism, 8*(2–3), 133–144.

UNDP-Laos. Lao PDR. Retrieved November 17, 2016, from http://www.la.undp.org/content/lao_pdr/en/home/countryinfo.html

Van Esterik, Penny. (2008). *Food culture in Southeast Asia.* Westport, CT: Greenwood Press.

World Food Programme. (2013). Food and nutrition atlas of Lao PDR. Retrieved November 5, 2016, from http://documents.wfp.org/stellent/groups/public/documents/ena/wfp260762.pdf

Vietnamese Cuisine

Vietnamese cuisine is known for balancing *âm* and *dương* (yin and yang) and composing ingredients, cooking methods, and flavors into the meal with rice as its basis. The cuisine reflects a complex and long history of influences from China, France, and neighboring countries of Southeast Asia, but retains unique and distinct foodways, methods of preparation, ingredients, and dishes.

Vietnamese cuisine is among the most distinctive, complex, and varied Asian kitchens. With rice as its staple, it features a huge array of ingredients, dishes, cooking techniques, and flavors concocted over three thousand years of recorded history and cultural elaboration. Although Vietnamese cuisine is shaped by its Southeast Asian ecology, the hard-working and resourceful Kinh (ethnic Vietnamese) have manipulated their habitat to such an extent that their environment, emerging produce, and foodways are the outcome of human efforts no less than the weather, topography, water, or soil. The foodways of immediate neighbors, most predominantly the Chinese, deeply influenced Vietnamese cuisine and had an impact in line with other cuisines, trade, immigration, colonialism, and other movements of people, ideas, and artifacts. The cuisine and customs of the French are perhaps the most notable of influences on contemporary Vietnamese cuisine.

One common misperception regarding Vietnamese cuisine is the idea that this is just a version of Chinese cuisine, or one form of Chinese regional cooking. Although the huge impact of Chinese foodways on Vietnamese cuisine cannot be denied, it possesses qualities, tendencies, and processes that make it unique and distinct from all other Asian kitchens.

Food Cosmology

Vietnamese cuisine was influenced by the East Asian cosmic model of *âm dương* (yin and yang), the two primordial forces from which everything in the world

57

was created. A balance between *âm* and *dương* is necessary in all things, while illness is caused by lack of balance between them, within a person, or between a person and the environment. Food plays an extremely important role in this scheme: health is maintained by a proper diet that maintains the balance between *âm* and *dương*, while illness is caused by an imbalance in the diet or food regime. In practice, these terms are translated into the binary of *nóng* (hot/warm) and *lạnh* (cold/cool) as foodstuffs, spices, and cooking techniques are attributed with heating or cooling qualities and are combined into dishes and meals so as to achieve or restore balance.

The second theoretical principle that structures Vietnamese foodways is that of the *ngũ hành* or "five elements" that make up the material and social universe. Just like *âm dương*, these elements require proper balance and are constantly adjusted so as to achieve harmony. The five elements (earth, water, wood, metal, and fire) are translated in the kitchen into rice, soup, greens, dry-cooked dishes, and fish sauce. Together, they make for a "proper dish" and a "proper meal," a well-balanced combination that most cooks tend to follow, though very few are aware of its theoretical grounds. This matrix is dynamic and flexible and can accommodate endless variations.

Rice

Rice is clearly the most important component in the Vietnamese cuisine—the *âm* substance that serves as the canvas over which the meal is drawn. The most common Vietnamese word for food, *cơm*, has the basic meaning of "cooked rice." Vietnamese has many words for rice, depending on whether it is husked or unhusked, cooked or uncooked, plain white rice or sticky (glutinous) rice. At most Vietnamese meals, a bowl filled with white rice sits in front of everyone present. Platters of food, sauces, and condiments are shared family-style, with small helpings added on top of the rice. If enough rice is available, several bowls of steamed white rice form the foundation of almost every meal. Fish, meat, and even vegetables are used mainly as condiments to be eaten with the rice. Without adequate rice, many people may leave a meal feeling hungry, even if other food was available.

When rice is scarce, people may add substantial amounts of corn, manioc, yams, or sweet potatoes to their diet to make their rice supply last longer. These foods are sometimes boiled and eaten separately and sometimes mixed in with the rice. But rice is almost always preferred. With certain dishes or for ceremonial offerings, glutinous rice is preferred. There are many kinds of both regular and sticky rice, depending on whether the grain is short or long, heavy or light. Ordinary rice is also pounded into powder to make different kinds of noodles and cakes, while glutinous rice is used for certain sweetmeats.

Fish and *Nước Mắm* (Fish Sauce)

Fish and other aquatic animals are the main source of animal protein. Most of the population is concentrated in river deltas and along the shores, and fishing in the ocean, rivers, canals, lakes, and rice fields is extensive. While large sea fish are most expensive and sought after, small fish, crab, shrimp, snail, eel, frogs, and many other small aquatic animals that live in shallow water are important elements of the daily diet.

The most common and important way of consuming fish, however, is in the form of *nước Mắm*, the ubiquitous fish sauce made of fermented long-jawed anchovy. *Nước mắm* is not only the most important source of animal protein and a variety of minerals in the Vietnamese diet, but also the defining element of the Vietnamese cuisine, used in virtually every Vietnamese dish (even coffee is roasted with fish sauce), making for their unique taste and aroma.

Most dishes are chopped into bite-sized pieces that are dipped into one or another of half a dozen common dipping sauces. The most prevalent of these is *nước chấm*, a sauce made from fish sauce mixed with crushed garlic, lime juice, sugar, and chili pepper, then slightly diluted with water. It is often served in individual dipping bowls, to which chili peppers can be added to taste.

Fresh Herbs and Vegetables

The third defining component of Vietnamese cuisine is fresh greens and herbs, crispy and aromatic, which are mixed with the rice, fish sauce, and other foods so as to create an endless variety of tastes, smells, and textures. These include lettuce and a variety of mints, basils, coriander, dill, bean sprouts, as well as unripe banana and star fruit. A unique form of consuming these herbs is in the form of *gỏi cuốn* or fresh spring rolls, made of rice paper rolls stuffed with greens and meat or seafood, and dipped in *nước chấm*.

Vegetables include spinach-like greens grown in water (*rau muống*) and many different kinds of beans, squash, pumpkins, cabbages, lettuce, eggplant, turnips, cucumbers, both regular and green onions, carrots, and tomatoes. These are eaten fresh, boiled, sautéed, or fried. Some are pickled, and some are dried for use in cooking. There are also many varieties of corn, yams, sweet potatoes, Western white potatoes, manioc, and other tuber crops. Peanut oil is the main cooking oil, and crushed peanuts are an important ingredient and taste agent. Đậu hũ (tofu), sữa đậu nành (soy milk), and soy sauce are important sources of vegetal protein.

Soups and Noodles

Soups and noodle dishes are also important parts of Vietnamese cuisine. Clear, light soups (canh) are routinely served with meals both in homes and in restaurants. In sophisticated settings, one can find wonton soup, eel soup, crab and asparagus soup, and many others.

Noodle soups are eaten at all hours of the day, as a meal or a snack. Most of these noodle dishes are commonly eaten in small restaurants or soup stands or purchased from sidewalk vendors. The most popular Vietnamese street dish is phở, which contains flat rice noodles in either beef broth or chicken broth with small amounts of meat. Another popular soup is made with a different kind of flat rice noodle (bún). Often this noodle is served in a bowl of broth containing grilled and seasoned meat (bún chả) or with snails (bún ốc). Another common soup is rice porridge (cháo), a rice gruel to which chicken, fish, pork, shrimp, organ meat (heart, liver), or eel may be added. Other soups are made with Chinese wheat noodles (mì), which are also sometimes served sautéed with vegetables, meat, or seafood.

Meat and Animal Products

Most Vietnamese eat rather little meat, and the meat eaten is mainly pork and chicken. People also eat meat from goats, ducks, and geese. Beef, introduced by the French, is scarce and expensive and is not often eaten. Beef flesh and bones, however, are crucial ingredients in one of Vietnam's most important dishes—phở bò, rice noodles served in beef stock. Another Vietnamese "classic" with strong French inclinations is bít tết or beefsteak.

Almost all parts of slaughtered animals are eaten, including organs, intestines, bones and skin. In the north, some people eat field rats and dogs, although the latter dish is usually preferred by older men. A few restaurants in and around major cities and resort areas specialize in snake meat; others serve exotic game dishes.

Chicken eggs are very common, and are consumed in large quantities. The terms ốp la (sunny side) and ốp lết (omelet), hint at French influence, especially in dishes such as bánh mì ốp la: a sizzling platter of sunny-side eggs served with meat balls and fresh baguette. Milk and dairy products are rarely consumed in Vietnam, with the exception of yoghurt (yaourt or sữa chua, literally "sour milk") and La Vache Qui Rit, a brand of processed cheese, both introduced by the French.

Beverages

Most Vietnamese drink large quantities of tea, usually warm green tea with nothing added. A thermos of hot water is often kept at the ready in homes and offices for making a pot of tea or topping up a pot that has cooled. Many varieties of tea are available: black, green, lotus, and jasmine. Tea bags can now be found in quite a few urban homes. Most Vietnamese men regularly drink coffee in coffee shops, a custom introduced by the French that has become an extremely important social institution. They tend to drink it very strong and sweet, usually by adding sweetened condensed milk. Limeade is also popular, and vendors sell juice from crushed sugarcane in the streets.

Alcoholic beverages are consumed in large quantities at social and ritualistic occasions, and quite a few elderly men are heavy drinkers. Locally distilled rice alcohol (*rượu gạo*) used to be the common and affordable drink, but nowadays beer, introduced by the French, is the drink of choice. Inexpensive, locally produced draft beer of variable quality is readily available in all cities and most towns. Canned and bottled beer, both domestic and imported, are very popular. Western-style wine made from grapes was once largely imported and expensive, but the quality of domestic wines has been improving. A growing but still small number of Vietnamese can now afford to buy an occasional bottle of wine or champagne. Many ethnic minority groups make wine from fermented rice or sometimes from manioc. Brandy is popular among those who drink hard liquor. Some people have developed a taste for imported scotch, bourbon, or blended whisky. Gin and vodka are less popular but are readily available in shops and stalls in major urban centers.

Fruits and Snacks

Vietnamese cuisine does not include the category of "dessert." Though a meal may end with tea and perhaps a little fruit, the sweet taste is an integral component of a well-balanced meal rather than an individual dish. Snacks in between mealtimes are popular. Many kinds kind of rice puddings or custards (*chè*) are sold by street vendors throughout the day. These usually contain glutinous rice, soybeans, black beans, green beans, tapioca, or lotus seeds. They don't usually contain milk products, but are made with plenty of sugar and one of a variety of flavorings such as ginger or sesame.

Fruits are abundant, affordable and popular. Common fruits include banana, papaya, mango, orange, lime, pomelo, tangerine, watermelon, jackfruit, lychee, rambutan, custard apple, jujube, persimmon, plum, dragon fruit, milk apple, star fruit, and mangosteen. Some Vietnamese like durian very much; others, not at all.

Local Specialties and Regional Cuisines

There are hundreds (and, according to some, thousands) of regional specialties, but some are common all over Vietnam. One of the best-known Vietnamese
dishes is the distinctive Vietnamese version of a spring roll, known as *nem* or
chả giò. Another dish, *cháo tôm*, is made by pounding shrimp, garlic, and other
ingredients into a paste and wrapping the paste around a thick stick of the inner portion of a sugarcane and then grilling it. *Bánh xèo* is something between
a pancake and an omelet. Ingredients include eggs, rice flour, coconut milk,
green onions, beans, and bean sprouts, fried in a hot skillet.

Fresh Spring Rolls

These fresh spring rolls (sometimes called summer
rolls) use rice paper to wrap vegetables, fresh herbs,
and, if desired, shrimp, marinated tofu or seitan, or
omelet strips. The beauty of these rolls is that they are
very flexible, and you can use whatever vegetables
or protein you have on hand, as long as you can cut
them into small, preferably long, pieces. They are
perfect to make in advance, and they hold for a day
or two in the refrigerator if wrapped in dampened
paper towels. They make a great lunch or light dinner
for hot summer days, when you don't want to turn on
the stove to cook. Serve with a dipping sauce, for

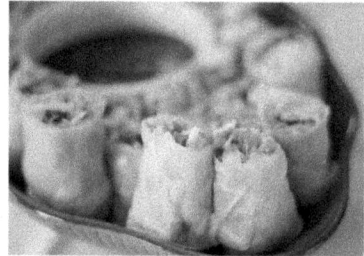

**Vietnamese spring rolls made
with rice wrappers.**

example, a simple one made with soy sauce, wine vinegar, a few drops of sesame oil, and
any spicy condiment of your choice.

Makes 10 to 15 rolls (depending on the size of the rice wrappers)

Ingredients
2½ ounces (70 g) thin rice noodles
2 tablespoons (30 ml) rice vinegar
1 tablespoon (15 ml) light soy sauce
1 head iceberg lettuce
1 cup (40 g) fresh herbs, such as mint leaves, basil leaves, cilantro leaves
¾ cup (75 g) shredded napa cabbage
½ cup (30 g) shredded or julienned carrot
½ cup (60 g) thinly sliced red bell pepper
¾ cup (75 g) bean sprouts
Round rice paper wrappers

▶▶

While essentially variations of a single dish, these local specialties feature specific qualities in accordance with local and regional food preferences and conventions. Food in the north tends to be somewhat fatty and bland, while the food in the center region is often spicy and salty, because in these poorer areas, smaller amounts of cooked food must flavor larger amounts of rice. For similar reasons, dishes in the center region tend to be smaller than those in the south. Southern cuisine is also sweeter than other regions.

There are hundreds of special dishes associated with a region, a city, or even a particular street. In Hanoi, a famous fish dish (*chả cá*) is associated with one small street, and shrimp cakes (*bánh tôm*) are sold mainly on a short strip along West Lake. Ho Chi Minh City cuisine features a marked French influence, which

---

Preparation

1. Prepare the noodles according to the package directions; usually this means soaking them in hot water for about 15 minutes. Drain the noodles and mix them with the vinegar and 1 tablespoon soy sauce. Set aside.

2. Remove the leaves from the lettuce and wash them, trying to keep them intact as much as possible. Prepare all other ingredients and lay them out so you can easily access them while assembling the rolls.

3. Fill a shallow bowl or deep plate with hot water. Keep more hot water at hand to refill if needed.

4. Soak a rice wrapper in hot water until it becomes soft and malleable, 30 to 45 seconds. Transfer to a plate or flat work surface.

5. Tear a piece of lettuce so it covers the surface of a narrow rectangle on the rice wrapper, leaving enough space on the sides to roll it up, and placing it just below the middle of the circle, with the long side facing toward you.

6. Top the lettuce with herbs, cabbage, carrots, bell peppers, bean sprouts, seasoned noodles, and shrimp or tofu, if you like.

7. To wrap the rolls, fold the bottom of the softened rice wrapper tightly over the filling. Hold in place while you fold the edges of the rice paper inward. Tightly roll the wrapper around the filling. Place on a plate with the seam side down.

8. Continue until you run out of one (or all) of your ingredients. (No worries if you run out of rice wrappers; the remaining ingredients make a fast and simple salad by simply tossing them together with a bit of dressing and some additional rice noodles).

9. Serve the rolls with a dipping sauce.

Source: Adapted by Marjolijn Kaiser from Katherine Polenz's *Vegetarian cooking at home* (2012).

can be discerned in dishes such as the sumptuous meal of "seven kinds of beef" *(thịt bò bảy món).*

The cuisine of Hue, former imperial capital and Buddhist headquarters, includes many varieties of distinctive cakes and dumplings and an astonishing variety of vegetarian dishes.

Nir AVIELI

Ben-Gurion University of the Negev

This article was adapted from an earlier version written by Neil L. JAMIESON, published in the *Encyclopedia of Modern Asia.*

Further Reading

Ngo, Bach. & Zimmerman, Gloria. (1979). *The classic cuisine of Vietnam.* Hauppauge, NY: Barron's Educational Series.

Nguyen, Luke. (2013). *The food of Vietnam.* Richmond, VC: Hardie Grant Books.

Nguyen, Luke, & Benson, Alan. (2011). *Indochine: baguettes and bánh mì: Finding France in Vietnam.* Sydney: Murdoch Books.

Routhier, Nicole, Jacobs, Martin, & Claiborne, Craig. (1989). *Foods of Vietnam.* New York: Stewart, Tabori, and Chang.

Trang, Corinne, & Hirsheimer, Christopher. (1999). *Authentic Vietnamese cooking: Food from a family table.* New York: Simon and Schuster.

Vu, Hong Lien. (2016). *Rice and baguette: A history of food in Vietnam.* Chicago: University of Chicago Press.

Indonesian Cuisine

The archipelago of Indonesia enjoys a unique and diverse cuisine famous for its bold, spicy flavors. Incorporating influences brought by traders from India, China, and the Middle East, along with native products and produce grown in its rich volcanic soil, the highlights of Indonesian cuisine include curries, as well as meat, vegetable, and tofu dishes accompanied by rice.

Indonesia, an archipelago composed of thousands of islands and hundreds of ethnic groups, is well known for its cuisine of distinct and diverse flavors. On the routes of commerce between India, China, and the Middle East, Indonesia developed a cuisine over time that reflects these foreign influences in its curries and stir-fries. In the basic Indonesian staples of rice (*nasi*) and vegetable dishes, fish, and occasionally beef or pork, the cuisine also reflects local products. Rice is grown in places with rich volcanic soil, either by terraced, wetland cultivation or by dry cultivation in eastern Indonesia.

The Wallace line, which separates the eco-regions of Asia and Australia, divides the Indonesian archipelago into two parts with distinctly different fauna and flora. The west consists of the larger islands of Sumatra, Java, Bali, and Kalimantan, while the east consists of Sulawesi, the Moluccas, the Lesser Sunda Islands, and West Papua. The differences in produce and cuisine roughly follow this biological division. Another dividing factor is the proximity to coastal areas, which are known for many fish and coconut dishes combined with spices and vegetables and complemented with tropical fruits.

Javanese, Sumatran, and Balinese cuisine represent the dominant Indonesian cuisines and are widely available across the archipelago because of inter-island migration. Beef *rendang*, a beef curry simmered in spices, chilies, and coconut until dry, originated in West Sumatra and is well known internationally. Together with *nasi goreng* (fried rice), *rendang* has become a café-style take-out food all over the world, found even in upmarket Asian restaurants in the Netherlands, the United States, and Australia. During the centuries before air travel, the mainly Muslim inhabitants of West Sumatra brought *rendang* with chilies and spices as preservatives on their long pilgrimages to Mecca.

Javanese *tempe* (tempeh) and *tahu* (tofu), both made from soybeans, form the basis of many Javanese dishes. While in the West these are often sold in health-food shops and specialty Asian groceries, they have become popular throughout Indonesia because of their high nutrition, low cost, easy storage, and delicious taste.

Eastern Indonesia (which is partly non-Muslim) and Bali also offers pork-based dishes, most notably Bali's *babi guling*, in which a pig is slow-roasted over an open fire on a hand-turned spit.

Beef Rendang

Beef rendang is a typical West Sumatran (Indonesia) dish and was originally made with buffalo meat. Although it is popular throughout Southeast Asia, this recipe comes from Singapore, and substitutes regular beef for the buffalo meat.

Ingredients
Spice Paste
16 dried red chilies, chopped
6 fresh red chilies, chopped
8 cloves garlic, chopped
One 3-inch (7.5 cm) piece of ginger, peeled and chopped
One 6-inch (15 cm) piece of galangal, peeled and chopped
10 candlenuts (or use macadamia nuts, almonds, or cashews), chopped
10 ounces (280 gr) onions, chopped
8 stalks lemongrass ·

Beef
10 tablespoons (70 g) grated unsweetened coconut (fresh or frozen)
4½ pounds (2 kg) beef chuck steak
TK vegetable oil
¾ teaspoon salt
¼ cup (50 g) palm sugar
2 tablespoons (16 g) ground coriander
4 stalks lemongrass, bruised
8 kaffir lime leaves
2 beef stock cubes
¼ cup (60 ml) tamarind juice (or 2 tablespoons [25 g] sugar and 2 tablespoons [30 ml] fresh lemon or lime juice)
2 tablespoons (30 ml) dark soy sauce
¼ cup (32 g) korma curry powder
¼ cup (60 ml) coconut milk

➤➤

Meals

In prosperous times, people in Indonesia expect to eat rice three times a day, accompanied by a main dish and side dishes. In Java, it is customary to offer to share food with others, and this practice has been adopted throughout Indonesia as a social gesture of inclusion. Guests arriving around mealtimes are invited to share in the food, with "*selamat makan*" or "enjoy your meal" said in the same way as "*bon appétit*." The food is placed on the table or floor mat where the diners serve themselves. In a middle-class home, a plate, spoon, and fork are used, while others may use banana leaves as plates and eat with their right hands.

Rice and a variety of dishes based on vegetables, fish, poultry, beef, pork, and pulses (beans) are cooked in a wok or a pot. The main ingredients are mixed, marinated, broiled, fried, or simmered with spices. Spices include pepper, nutmeg, coriander, lesser galingale, turmeric, candlenuts (*kemiri*, similar to a macadamia nut), garlic, onions, and chilies, which are crushed using pestle and mortar. During feasts, such as weddings and Lebaran (the Muslim

---

Preparation

1. To make the spice paste, mix all ingredients in a food processor or blender to a smooth paste. Set aside.

2. To prepare the beef, fry the grated coconut in a dry pan (without oil) until slightly browned, then transfer it to a food processor and process it to a coarse powder.

3. Bring a large pot of water to a boil. Place the beef briefly in the boiling water, swirling just until the meat changes color. Remove the beef and cut it into cubes.

4. In a deep skillet or wok, fry the spice paste over medium heat in a layer of vegetable oil and add the salt. After about 3 minutes, add the palm sugar and ground coriander and fry for another 2 minutes.

5. Add the bruised lemongrass and fry it with the spice paste for approximately 10 minutes.

6. Add the beef and lime leaves to the fried spice paste. Fry the beef until it is browned.

7. Add just enough water to cover the meat; add the beef stock cubes. Stir in the tamarind juice, dark soy sauce, and curry powder. Cover and simmer over very low heat for approximately 3 hours, until the beef is tender.

8. Add the coconut milk and bring to a gentle boil. Turn off the heat and stir in the coarse coconut powder.

Source: Mrs. Lim Lorna Hwang

celebration at the end of the fasting month of Ramadan), a variety of dishes are served: for instance, yellow (turmeric) rice accompanied by fried chicken, fried fish, chicken curry, or prawn curry and garnished with thinly sliced omelets and greens. This combination is the basis of the internationally acclaimed *rijst-tafel* (rice and a set of special dishes), a Dutch colonial's gastronomic adaptation of the typical East Indies (as Indonesia used to be known) feast.

Everyday cooking relies on vegetables available daily in the market, such as cabbage, *kang-kung* (a kind of watercress), Chinese cabbage, snake beans, a variety of bean sprouts, and marrows. *Gado-gado*, a famous Indonesian vegetarian dish, consists of vegetables, including tomatoes, garnished with thinly sliced boiled eggs and crushed *krupuk* (prawn crackers), and complemented with peanut sauce as a dressing. This low-cost but healthy dish is popularly eaten as a snack or main meal during mid-day, competing with chicken *satay* (cubed meat on a skewer), both of which are available in street food stalls or from hawkers and restaurants.

Sweets and Beverages

Indonesians eat sweets as snacks, not as desserts. Dessert is commonly a selection of tropical fruits in season, particularly bananas, which are available all year. Cakes, puddings, biscuits, and pastries have been much influenced by the Dutch, while traditional sweets are made of cassavas, sweet potatoes, glutinous rice, palm sugar, or grated coconut, or a combination of these. The mainly Muslim population does not drink alcohol with meals; however, for feasts and special occasions in some areas, people may drink a locally produced fermented palm wine known as *tuak, moke* (palm wine from the *lontar* palm), *arak* (distilled liquor from sugar palm), or *brem* (fermented rice). People usually drink hot or iced tea or water with their meals.

Today, Indonesian cuisine also reflects the Western influence of fast foods such as breads and hamburgers and the Chinese influence of noodles, along with the traditional foods based on fresh tropical produce with various tastes: spicy, sweet, savory, sour, or pungent. The home of a wide range of spices, Indonesia became famous during three and a half centuries of colonial rule for these condiments and since then for its cuisine.

Catharina Purwani WILLIAMS

Further Reading

Brackman, Agnes de Keizer, & Brackman, Cathay. (2015). *The complete Indonesian cookbook*. New York: Cavendish Square Publishing.

Freedman, Paul, & Koo Siu Ling. (2015). *Culture, cuisine, cooking: an East Java Peranakan memoir.* Eindhoven, The Netherlands: Lecturis.

Handoyo, Crisfella Cokrro, *et al.* (2017). Klappertaart: An Indonesian - Dutch influenced traditional food. *JEF Journal of Ethnic Foods.*

Hiang, M., & Djalil, Roos. (1995). *Indonesian dishes and desserts.* Jakarta, Indonesia: Gaya Favorit Press.

Hutton, Wendy. (1999). *The Food Of Bali: Authentic recipes from the islands of the gods.* North Clarendon, VT: Tuttle Publishing.

Jákl, Jiří. (2015). Bhoma's kitchen: Food culture and food symbolism in pre-Islamic Java. *Global Food History Global Food History, 1*(1), 33–57.

Kruger, Vivienne L. (2014). *Balinese food: exploring the traditional cuisine and food culture of Bali.* North Clarendon, VT: Tuttle Publishing.

Marks, Copeland. (1994). *The exotic kitchens of Indonesia: Recipes from the outer islands.* New York: M. Evans and Company.

Ministry of Tourism and Creative Economy, Republic of Indonesia. (2012). *Taste the Indonesian cuisine.* Jakarta.

Owen, Sri. (1987). Indonesian Cuisine - at its best. *New Home Economics, 33*(5), 5–7.

Owen, Sri. (1995). *Indonesian regional cooking.* New York: St. Martin Press.

Reid, Anthony. (1988). *Southeast Asia in the age of commerce, 1450–1680: The lands below the winds* (vol. 1). New Haven, CT: Yale University Press.

Situngkir, Hokky; Maulana, Ardian: & Mauludy, Rolan. (2015). A portrait of diversity in Indonesian traditional cuisine. *SSRN Journal SSRN Electronic Journal.*

Spierings, Thea, & van Teeffelen, Marnix. (2009). *The real taste of Indonesia: a culinary journey: 100 unique family recipes.* Melbourne: Hardie Grant Books.

Van der Kroef, Justus M. (1952). Rice legends of Indonesia. *Jamerfolk: The Journal of American Folklore, 65*(255), 49–55.

Von Holzen, Heinz. (2005). *Feast of flavours from the Balinese kitchen: A step-by-step culinary adventure.* Singapore: Marshall Cavendish Cuisine.

Von Holzen, Heinz. (2007). *Bali unveiled: the secrets of Balinese cuisine.* Singapore: Marshall Cavendish Cuisine.

Von Holzen, Heinz. (2010). *Street foods of Bali.* Singapore: Marshall Cavendish Cuisine.

Von Holzen, Heinz. (2015). *The little Indonesian cookbook.* Singapore: Marshall Cavendish International (Asia).

Yuen, Dina, & Chu, Glenn. (2012). *Indonesian cooking: satays, sambals and more : 81 homestyle recipes with the true taste of Indonesia.* Clarendon, VT: Tuttle Publishing.

Malaysian Cuisine

Malaysian cuisine is infused with a variety of influences from centuries of immigrants, traders, and colonial powers who arrived from both East and West. Chinese and Indian immigrants have left the most lasting impression on the gastronomy of this region, and the liberal use of spices and herbs makes for one of the most popular and flavorful cuisines in Asia.

Malaysian cuisine reflects the rich multicultural heritage of this Southeast Asian nation. When the port sultanate of Malacca (1400–1511) was founded, it attracted traders from both the East and West. Later, culinary traditions were brought by Portuguese (1511–1641), Dutch (1641–1824), and English (1876–1957) colonists, as well as merchants from China, India, Saudi Arabia, and the Indonesian Archipelago.

The dietary staples of rice and noodles reflect in part geography and native plant life, while the spice trade left an indelible impression on present-day tastes. The cuisines of Malaysia's three main ethnic groups, the Malays, Chinese, and Indians, form the core of Malaysian cuisine today.

Various manifestations of rice dishes abound, and accompanying dishes are highly spiced in traditional Malay cuisine, with many homes chefs grinding their own fresh herbs and spices such as anise seed, fenugreek, and cumin. Other favorites include coriander, turmeric, and candlenut (which helps to thicken sauces). Fresh chilies are always used, as well as ginger, shallots, and garlic. *Belacan*, a fermented shrimp paste, is a quintessential ingredient; it is toasted and used to provide a depth of flavor to curries and *sambal* (a spicy chili-pepper-based paste). Coconut cream features prominently in many dishes, while the oil of the coconut is used for cooking, and the sap of the flower is made into unrefined palm sugar, known as *gula melaka*, which imparts a deep caramel flavor to desserts.

Malay food is ever-evolving as old recipes for curries, *sambals*, and chutneys (spicy fruit- or vegetable-based pastes) reappear. The best-known examples of Malay cuisine are *satay,* meat kebabs served with a spicy peanut sauce,

70

Compressed Rice
Lontong

In *The Rice Book*, author Sri Owen explains that "compressed rice (*lontong*) is always eaten cold; served with satay, for example, it soaks up the hot sauce, and its coolness and soft texture contrast with the hot spices and the meat. In Indonesia and Malaysia, the rice is cooked in a cylinder of banana leaf or in a little woven packet of coconut fronds, in which case it is called *ketupat*." Since most people outside those countries won't have the more exotic packaging material at hand, Owen suggest simply using aluminum foil or a bag made of muslin or heatproof perforated paper. "Boil-in-the-bag rice ought to be ideal, and the bags themselves are indeed excellent. Unfortunately, almost all boil-in-the-bag rice nowadays is parboiled, and this makes it useless for *lontong* because the grains cannot compress and merge together." Make the bags for this recipe about 6 inches (15 cm) square bags, using muslin or heatproof perforated paper.

Serves 8 to 10

Ingredients
1 cup (200 g) long-grain rice, preferably basmati or jasmin, washed and drained
7½ cups (1.8 L) hot water, plus more as needed
Pinch of salt

Preparation
1. Fill each muslin bag one-third full with rice. Close up the opening. Combine the water and salt in a large pot and bring to a boil. When it reaches boiling, put in the bags of rice and let the water simmer gently for about 1 hour 15 minutes. The bags of rice must always be submerged, so add more boiling water as required during cooking.

2. Take out the bags and drain them in a colander. When they are cold, refrigerate them until use.

3. To serve, remove the bags and cut up the "cushions" into 1-inch (2.5 cm) chunks or slices using a sharp knife dipped in water.

Source: Sri Owen. (1994). *The rice book: The definitive book on rice, with hundreds of exotic recipes from around the world*. New York: St. Martin's Press.

cucumbers, onions, and rice cooked in coconut fronds; *nasi lemak,* rice cooked in coconut cream and served with a hard-boiled egg, fried chicken, and various condiments; and char kway teow, a Chinese-inspired dish of stir-fried rice noodles with prawns, eggs, bean sprouts, and chives.

Chinese traders have been travelling and settling in Malaysia since the fifteenth century. Today, Malaysian Chinese cuisine can be categorized as Cantonese, Hainanese, Hakka, or Hokkien, reflecting the different regions in south China where these traders originated. Again, rice and noodles are staples in the offerings of one-dish meals. Seafood is favored, vegetables as well as meats are often served with rice, and noodles are prepared in many different ways. Most notable is the hawker fare of Penang, located in the northwest of Peninsular Malaysia, as well as the fusion Nonya cuisine of the Chinese Peranakans (descendants of traders who wed local Malay women) who settled there and in Malacca. Cantonese offerings can be found farther south in the Klang Valley, situated in the state of Selangor, and in the city of Ipoh in the state of Perak.

Indian food, contrary to popular belief, is not always spicy. Vegetarian offerings are plentiful in Malaysian Indian cuisine, and the most popular dishes include rice with various curries served on a section of banana leaf, in South Indian style. Indian-style breads are numerous, among them *roti canai* (the local name for *paratha,* a crispy bread with several thin layers), *chapati* (a thicker whole-wheat bread), and *thosai* (a thin pancake made from the paste of ground lentils and rice). The style of preparation of accompanying dishes differs according to India's various regions and states, and there are distinctions between Indian Muslim and South Indian cuisines.

Malaysians enjoy a wide variety of tropical fruits, most notably the malodorous durian and the mangosteen, called the queen of fruit for its position secondary to the durian. Desserts are often bought from local bakeries or enjoyed at hawker stalls, as they are intricate to make. These include *sago gula Melaka,* sago pudding with palm sugar and coconut milk; *kuih Nyonya,* small delicate cakes with coconut and a variety of other ingredients; and *bubur cha cha,* a warm concoction of sago, cubes of sweet potato, and the ubiquitous coconut milk.

Mark Stephan FELIX

Mahidol University, Thailand

Further Reading

Faizah Omar; Abisheganaden, Hanna; Ellina Majid; & Ayesha Harben. (2000). *Traditional Malay cuisine: A rich selection in culinary heritage.* Kuala Lumpur: Berita

Hutton, Wendy. (Ed.). (1995). *The food of Malaysia: Authentic recipes from the crossroads of Asia.* Singapore: Periplus Editions.

Leinbach, T. R. & Ulack. R. (2000). *South East Asia diversity and development.* Upper Saddle River, NJ: Prentice-Hall.

Malaysian festival cuisine. (1995). Kuala Lumpur, Malaysia: Berita.

Marks, C. (1997). *The exotic kitchens of Malaysia.* New York: Donald I. Fine Books.

Traditional Malaysian cuisine. (1983). Kuala Lumpur, Malaysia: Berita.

Pawanchik, Azza . (2008). *Makan: introduction to modern Malaysian food.* Shah Alam: Kumpulan Karangkraf.

Singaporean Cuisine

The cuisine of Singapore reflects a history of colonization, immigration, and the intermingling of neighboring cultures in Southeast Asia. Influenced primarily by Malay, Chinese, and Indian cuisines, the local fare of Singapore is complex, flavorful, and eclectic. The passion that Singaporeans bring to this aspect of their culture has helped to make the island one of the world's premier food destinations.

Singapore, located at the southern tip of the Malay Peninsula in Southeast Asia, was already a flourishing trading port by the fourteenth century. The colonial port city of Singapore was established with the arrival of the British in the 1820s. With its entrepot trade status, it attracted immigrants from China, India, and other parts of Asia. It is the aggregation of these diverse groups that has contributed to the richness of Singaporean cuisine.

History

The British ruled over Singapore for more than 120 years but left few significant culinary legacies in the everyday life of Singaporeans today. A handful of British colonial dishes like curries, kedgeree, mulligatawny, and the Sunday tiffin (a multi-dish buffet lunch) are but infrequent reminders in nostalgia-themed restaurants or hotels. These are hybrid dishes of British and Asian elements, however, and were created by Asian cooks.

In the intervening years of Japanese occupation in World War II, between 1942 and 1945, tapioca and sweet potatoes were staples that defined the hardships endured by Singaporeans. This was the only period in Singapore's modern history when there were widespread food shortages.

Malay Food

Malay food is derived from a blend of cultures from China, India, Indonesia, the Middle East, and Europe. Rice is the staple and is supplemented by many coconut-based dishes, chilies, and other spices. The prominent use of rhizomes and bulbs like galangal, ginger, and turmeric as well as lemon grass, coriander, screw pine leaf, and curry leaf underscore the importance of fragrance in Malay cooking. These aromatics add flavor and fragrance to the different kinds of

---

Satay

Popular around Southeast Asia, satays are meat kebabs served with a spicy peanut sauce.

Serves 4 to 6

Ingredients
2 pounds (900 g) boneless chicken breasts, beef, or pork

Marinade
⅓ cup (75 ml) honey
½ cup (120 ml) water
Juice and pulp of 1 lime
2½ tablespoons (20 g) ground coriander
1½ teaspoons (9 g) salt
2 stalks fresh lemongrass, or 2 teaspoons (2 g) dried lemongrass
2 ounces (56 g) galangal (or ginger), peeled
1 fresh red chili
1 large onion, peeled
¼ cup (60 ml) vegetable oil

Peanut Sauce
1 stalk lemongrass, or 1 teaspoon (1 g) dried lemongrass
½ ounce (14 g) galangal (or ginger), peeled
8 dried Thai chilies, soaked in warm water, drained
3 cloves garlic
¼ onion, peeled
¼ cup (60 ml) vegetable oil
1 cup (150 g) toasted peanuts, finely ground in a coffee mill or with a mortar and pestle
2 teaspoons (10 ml) rice vinegar
¼ cup (60 ml) honey
¼ cup (60 ml) fresh lime juice
2 cups (480 ml) water
¾ teaspoon (4.5 g) salt

▶▶

curries and other dishes. Further, cinnamon, cloves, nutmeg, and mace are the foundation of many Malay spice mixes. Fried shallots and garlic add depth, while spiciness comes from both fresh and dried chilies. Dried shrimp paste provides the umami taste, while coconut milk and palm sugar lend sweetness, and tamarind and lime juice add tartness and fragrance. Malay classic dishes include different kinds of curries like *rendang* (a "dry" curry with origins in Indonesia) and *korma* (a South Asian dish with a thick sauce that includes yoghurt or cream), using beef, mutton, chicken, fish, or prawns. The highlight of Malay cuisine is satay, thought to have derived from the Arab kebab. The meat is thinly sliced, threaded on bamboo skewers, grilled over coals, and served with a peanut sauce.

Ethnic Influences

The island city-state of Singapore is dwarfed by its nearest neighbor, Peninsular Malaysia, both in landmass and population figures, but they are forever linked by similarities in social and cultural mores and most discernibly in similar food-ways. Indeed, there are those who doubt whether a uniquely Singaporean cuisine exists. In practical terms, the multicultural make-up of Malaysia and Singapore are similar, with the major races of Chinese, Indian, Malay, and other

---

Preparation

1. Cut the meat into ½-inch (1.3 cm) cubes.

2. Thread the meat on skewers and spread them out in a shallow pan. Set aside.

3. To make the marinade, heat the honey and water in a small saucepan over low heat. Add the lime juice and pulp, coriander, and salt; stir and set aside. In a food processor or blender, grind the lemongrass, galangal, chili, onion, and oil; add the wet ingredients. Stir well, then pour over the skewered meat and marinate for at least 6 hours.

4. To make the peanut sauce, puree the lemongrass, galangal, chilies, garlic, and onion in a food processor or blender. Heat the oil in a skillet, then add the spicy mixture, cooking for 1 minute, until fragrant. Add the remaining ingredients and boil the mixture, stirring often, for 15 minutes, or until the sauce becomes creamy.

5. Grill the marinated, skewered meat until cooked through. Serve with the spicy peanut sauce as a dip.

Source: This recipe comes courtesy of the Singapore Tourism Board and Singapore chef Violet Oon, adapted from Mother Earth Living's website (https://www.motherearthliving.com/Cooking-Methods/Spice-Island-Singapore-Satay).

minority groups. Most of the dishes consumed in the two countries are familiar and recognizable to the people of both nations. Differences could be as subtle as the variation of sweetness or spiciness for any particular dish for the two countries.

Food in Singapore has been an important site for history-making and nation-building and also as a marketing tool in efforts to make the country into a food destination by the tourism board. Singapore's mix of racial and ethnic diversity, along with its corresponding culinary offerings, have been touted towards this end. The food cultures of Chinese, Malays, and Indians present a bewildering smorgasbord of distinct dishes from each community.

Most of the regional cooking traditions and dialect groups (Hokkien, Cantonese, Teochew, Hainanese, and Hakka) in China are represented in Singapore. Fine-dining restaurants from the north and east feature dishes from Beijing and Shanghai. Casual eating outlets and home-cooking also replicate dishes from the northern and eastern regions. Cantonese cuisine, universally known to be synonymous with Chinese cuisine outside China, is prominent in Singapore too. Most of the Cantonese restaurants follow Hong Kong traditions. Cantonese-style roasts such as suckling pig, roast pork, and roast duck are easily obtainable for takeaway meals as well as from restaurants. The *dim sum* breakfast or lunch, where small dishes are served with tea, is widely available in Singapore. The largest dialect group, the Hokkiens, are well known for hearty pork-braised dishes, usually eaten with steamed buns. Hakka dishes are similarly robust. Teochew cooking is lighter and uses more seafood. Hainanese were hired as cooks in colonial households and are also well-known for operating coffee shops. Their distinct brew of coffee uses Robusta beans roasted with sugar and butter for intense flavor and aroma.

Indian Influences

Most of the early Indian arrivals to Singapore were recruited by the British, and they were instrumental in introducing ingredients and dishes from South Asia to the city. Dishes and recipes change as they travel, and Indian food in Singapore took on ingredients and methods of cooking from other cultures so that new dishes emerged. Fish head curry, for instance, is such a dish and has become the signature feature of an Indian meal in Singapore. The different kinds of curries that exist in Singapore today are as much a story of its colonization as its Indian migrant history. The curries that the British consumed were of the Anglo-Indian variety, similar to those concocted by servants in colonial India. Often, adding a tablespoon of curry powder is sufficient to call a dish a curry. Singaporeans, however, generally buy fresh curry pastes from Indian stalls and have different combinations of spices made up for particular meat, chicken, or seafood curries.

Eurasian and Peranakan Influences

Mixed marriages, or the cohabitation of local women with immigrants or colonialists, gave rise to Eurasian and Peranakan cultures and cuisines. Eurasians, of Asian and Portuguese, Dutch, or British heritage, developed their own culture and identity. Features of their kitchens include the essential pastes of chili paste and *rempahs* (ground herbs and spices in a paste) that go into the making of unique meals that are a combination of European and Asian ingredients and cooking methods. The Peranakans are understood to be the mixed cultures of two racial groups (between Chinese and Malays, for instance) with a distinct hybridized cuisine. Peranakan Chinese are known for combining pungent and aromatic roots, herbs, and spices from Malay cooking traditions with other ingredients of Chinese origin. Another aspect of this cuisine is the use of souring agents such as green mango, *belimbing* (*Averrhoa bilimbi*), and pineapple.

Finally, there are crossovers of cuisines from the different cultures in Singapore. The hybridity in Malay cuisine and the Islamization of Chinese food as well as the hybridization of Indian food are evident in dishes offered in food courts and restaurants. Ingredients or cooking methods are borrowed from other cultures and served as distinct creole dishes.

Cecilia LEONG-SALOBIR

University of Wollongong

Further Reading

Duruz, Jean, & Gaik Cheng Khoo. (2015). *Eating together: Food, space, and identity in Malaysia and Singapore.* Lanham, NC: Rowman & Littlefield.

Leong-Salobir, Cecilia. (2011). *Food culture in Colonial Asia: A taste of empire.* London: Routledge.

Leong-Salobir, Cecilia. (2011). Food stories: Culinary links of an island state and a continent.

In Ian Austin (Ed.), *Australia-Singapore relations: Successful bilateral relations in a*

historical and contemporary context. Singapore: Select Books & Edith Cowan

University.

Tarulevicz, Nicole. (2013). *Eating her curries and kway: A cultural history of food in Singapore.* Champaign: University of Illinois Press.

Wong Hong Suen. (2009). *Wartime kitchen: Food and eating in Singapore 1942–1950.* Singapore: National Museum of Singapore.

Philippine Cuisine

The cuisine of the Philippines combines flavors of its neighbors in China and Southeast Asia with indigenous preferences and influences from centuries of colonial rule by Spain. Most prevalent are fish, rice, and coconut-infused dishes, often with a sour-salty flavor.

The cuisine of the Philippines reflects its Southeast Asian location, its proximity to China, as well as its complex history of colonization, which includes more than three hundred years of Spanish rule, beginning in 1521, and fifty years of American dominance. Combined with these influences is a history of commerce with Chinese and Malay neighbors. These circumstances have made the Philippines one of the "centers for gastronomic change" (Sokolov 1991, 14–25).

The result is a dynamic cuisine in which no one dish can properly represent the country. *Sinigang*, a broth of fish or shrimp paired with vegetables and flavored with tamarind, guava, or citrus fruits, may be the most indigenous dish, and one which best symbolizes the sour-salty combination preferred by Filipinos. *Adobo*, made with chicken or pork cooked in vinegar and garlic, originates in Mexican-Spanish influences, while *pancit* (noodles crowned with meat, vegetables, or local ingredients) and *lumpia*, a spring roll fried or served fresh, derive from Chinese cuisine.

Composed of seven thousand islands, the Philippines is surrounded by the sea. Fresh seafood is a must, especially in *kinilaw*, a dish similar to ceviche in which fresh fish is marinated in vinegar and immediately eaten. Fish and a jar of palm wine were the first gifts to greet the Portuguese explorer Ferdinand Magellan and his party. Today, fish served with rice is a Filipino meal boiled down to its essence. There are at least 160 words relating to rice and its prominent role as the staple grain, although in some areas corn or sweet potatoes are preferred. Beloved for its versatility, rice not only makes a meal but is used for rice cakes called *puto* as well as numerous sweets. The coconut is a close second to rice; its juice and meat are consumed fresh or used to flavor cooking, while

78

Garlic Fried Rice

Sinangag

Unlike in the West, breakfast in Asia often contains savory dishes, including rice, pickled vegetables, steamed buns, and even noodles. In the Philippines, a favorite breakfast item is *sinangag*, or garlic fried rice. It uses the rice left over from the previous evening, which is fried and served with crispy baked garlic. It can be served with scrambled or fried eggs, and sometimes other vegetables, seafood, or meat is added.

Serves 4

Ingredients
4 cups (800 g) cold cooked white rice
¼ cup (60 ml) plus 2 tablespoons (30 ml) cooking oil
4 cloves garlic, minced
Sea salt and ground black pepper

Preparation
1. Break the cold rice into separate grains.

2. Heat the quarter cup (60 ml) oil in a small pan over low heat. Add the garlic and cook until golden brown, 7 to 10 minutes, stirring occasionally. Remove the garlic from the pan and drain it on paper towels.

3. Heat 2 tablespoons oil (30 ml) in a wok or heavy-bottomed skillet over high heat. Add the rice and stir constantly for about 3 minutes, until the rice is heated through.

4. Add the garlic and mix well. Season with salt and pepper.

Source: Inspired by recipes from https://www.kawalingpinoy.com/sinangag/ and http://panlasangpinoy.com/2014/07/30/sinangag-recipe/.

the heart of the tree is enjoyed as a delicacy. Reliance on nature is another trademark of Philippine cuisine, seen in the use of cooking utensils that flavor food. The hollow of a bamboo pole can be made to boil rice, while banana leaves can steam fish or meat as well as flavor *bibingka* (rice cakes topped with sugar and native cheese).

Regional Specialties

Each province or region is known for its specialties. In Pampanga, a province reputed to harbor good cooks, cured meats are among the specialties. *Tocino* is made from thin slices of seasoned pork and served with eggs over fried rice for breakfast, or sometimes it is *longanisa*, a slightly spicy and sweet pork sausage. *Pinakbet*, a vegetable dish of bitter melon, eggplant, and *bagoong* (a popular condiment made from fermented tiny shrimp or anchovies) typifies Ilocano foodways. Down south, in Muslim Mindanao and Sulu, pork is avoided. Instead, goat, beef, and seafood cooked with coconut milk and spicy red chilies are favored.

Fiestas and special occasions like Christmas call for rich Spanish-based dishes, such as *lechon* (roasted pig), *paella* (saffron-flavored rice seasoned with tomatoes and garlic and topped with meats and seafood), and chicken or fish *relleno* (stuffed chicken or fish), with *leche flan* (an egg custard) for dessert. For everyday meals, the lower and middle classes prefer Malay- and Chinese-influenced dishes. *Merienda* is the afternoon snack, as simple as a mango fruit or as elaborate as *puto* and *dinuguan* (pork blood stew). Favorite *pulutan* or snacks, like fertilized duck eggs called *balut*, are both street food as well as snacks eaten during drinking sessions, and are believed to be an aphrodisiac for men. Despite foreign influences, the liberal use of flavoring condiments like *bagoong*, chilies, crushed garlic, and vinegar can be said to indigenize Filipino cuisine, making dishes unique to that country.

Margaret C. MAGAT

SpecPro Professional Services (SPS)

Further Reading

Aranas, Jennifer; Briggs, Brian; & Lande, Michael. (2006). *The Filipino-American kitchen: Traditional recipes, contemporary flavors.* New York: Tuttle Publishing.

Barreto, Glenda Rosales, & Fenix, Michaela. (2013). *Kulinarya: A guidebook to Philippine cuisine.* Mandaluyong City, Philippines: Anvil Publishing.

Basan, Ghillie. (2015). *Classic recipes of the Philippines: Traditional food and cooking in 25 authentic dishes.* Leicester, UK: Lorenz Books.

Basan, Ghillie, & Laus, Vilma. (2011). *A taste of the Philippines: Classic Filipino recipes made easy, with 70 authentic traditional dishes shown step by step in more than 400 beautiful photographs.* Leicester, UK: Southwater Publishing.

Besa, Amy; Dorotan, Romy; & Oshima, Neil. (2012). *Memories of Philippine kitchens: stories and recipes from far and near.* New York: Stewart, Tabori & Chang.

Comsti, Angelo. (2015). *Fuss-free Filipino food: Quick & easy dishes for everyday cooking.* Singapore: Marshall Cavendish International (Asia).

Comsti, Angelo; Tham, Melissa; & Maculangan, At. (2014). *The Filipino family cookbook: Recipes and stories from our home kitchen.* Singapore: Marshall Cavendish International (Asia).

Diego, Arlene. (2008). *Feast of flavours from the Philipino kitchen: a step-by-step culinary adventure.* Singapore: Marshall Cavendish Cuisine.

Fernandez, Doreen. (1994). *Tikim: Essays on Philippine food and culture.* Pasig, Philippines: Anvil Publishing.

Fernandez, Doreen, & Alegre, Edilberto. (1988). *Sarap: Essays on Philippine food.* Manila, Philippines: Mr. & Mrs. Publishing.

Fernandez, Doreen, & Alegre, Edilberto. (1991) *Kinilaw: A Philippine cuisine of freshness.* Makati, Philippines: Bookmark.

Fernandez, Doreen, & Best, Jonathan. (2000). *Palayok: Philippine food through time, on site, in the pot.* Makati City, Philippines: Bookmark.

Lopez, Mellie. (1984). *A study of Philippine folklore.* Ph.D. diss. University of California, Berkeley.

Sokolov, Raymond. (1991). *Why we eat what we eat: How the encounter between the New World and the Old changed the way everyone on the planet eats.* New York: Summit Books.

Gapultos, Marvin. (2013). *The adobo road cookbook a Filipino food journey.* Tokyo: Tuttle Publishing.

Newman, Yasmin. (2013). *7000 islands: A food portrait of the Philippines.* Australia: Hardie Grant Books.

O'Boyle, Lily Gamboa. (1993). *Pacific crossings: The new Philippine cuisine.* New York: Acacia Corp.

Reyes, Cid. (2009). *Pinoy umami: The heart of Philippine cuisine.* Makati City, Philippines: Ajinomoto Philippines Corp.

Tabura, Adam, & Tanabe, Kaz. (2016). *A Filipino kitchen: Traditional recipes with an island twist.* Honolulu: Mutual Publishing.

Central and West Asia

Central Asian Cuisines

The cuisines of Central Asia share many components, dishes, and methods of preparation, while their differences reflect the nomadic lifestyle of some peoples or the agriculture-based economies of others. An often harsh and arid climate also plays a role and is shown in the reliance on meat and cultured dairy products.

Central Asian cuisine encompasses the traditional culinary practices of the region's five countries, whose methods of food preparation can be divided into two groups. Historically, Kazakhstan and Kyrgyzstan were populated primarily by nomadic peoples, who for centuries herded sheep, camels, and horses. Their constant movement left no time for agriculture or complex cooking; the people of these countries relied mainly on the meat and milk provided by their herds, with very little else to diversify their diet. In contrast, inhabitants of the more settled regions of Uzbekistan, Tajikistan, and Turkmenistan cultivated crops and developed sophisticated cooking techniques, thanks to greater availability of produce as well as their ability to spend time at the hearth.

Central Asia's largely harsh and arid climate meant that even in the agricultural regions people relied heavily on meat and cultured dairy products, with relatively few vegetables beyond hardy root crops. Beginning in the late nineteenth century, however, many new crops were introduced, and as the traditional nomadic way of life began to disappear, more garden crops were sown, a process accelerated by the use of widespread irrigation during the Soviet period. Today, after more than a century of change and outside influence, the differences among the Central Asian countries are far less pronounced than they once were, and it is possible to make certain generalizations about the foods of the region.

Ingredients

The ingredients of Central Asian cuisines share many similarities, though the terms and uses may vary from country to country. Most prevalent are the importance of meat and cultured dairy products, and the love of flatbreads and pilafs.

MEATS AND MEAT DISHES

Meat remains an important food source throughout Central Asia. Lamb is the most popular, although the Turkmens favor mountain goat or kid, while Kazakhs are partial to organ meats. The Kyrgyz consider horsemeat sausage a delicacy. The two most widespread methods for preparing meat are grilling and boiling (or steaming). Uzbekistan is renowned for its many varieties of kebab (skewered grilled meat, either in whole pieces or ground). The excellent *kiyma* kebab is made by shaping seasoned ground lamb around a skewer.

Turkmen and Tajik meat cookery also depends on the grill, but in Kazakhstan and Kyrgyzstan boiled meats are more common. An ancient dish still eaten today is *kavurdak,* meat that has been stewed in its own fat and then stored in vessels for long keeping. Meat is also preserved by drying it on tall poles in the sun. Both methods reflect the necessities of itinerant life.

Meat is used to flavor a variety of soups; especially prized is the *lagman* found throughout Central Asia, a hearty soup of lamb, carrots, and noodles. Unlike many clear European and Asian soups, the soups of Central Asia are nearly always stew-like, enriched with thickeners like potatoes, chickpeas, or mung beans. These soups tend to be rich and filling from the addition of the prized fat from fat-tailed sheep.

Domestic fowl is not as popular as red meat; more highly appreciated are wild fowl such as pheasant and quail. Since pork is proscribed under Islamic law, it is consumed solely by the minority non-Muslim populations. Fish is regularly eaten only in regions that have a significant water source, such as western Turkmenistan and Kazakhstan bordering on the Caspian Sea.

DAIRY PRODUCTS

The second most important component of Central Asian cuisine is the wide array of cultured dairy products made from the milk of sheep and camels and, to a lesser extent, goats and cows. These include *koumiss* (slightly fermented milk), *ayran* (yoghurt mixed with water), *kaymak* (clotted cream), and *suzma* (yoghurt cheese). Uzbek cuisine in particular boasts numerous milk-based soups, one of the best being *shirkovok* (milk soup with pumpkin and rice). Eggs are not significant in Central Asian cookery.

GRAINS, LEGUMES, AND BREADS

Central Asian cuisine is perhaps best known for its extensive variety of rice pilafs (*palov*). Uzbekistan alone is said to have one hundred different types, and their proper preparation is considered an art. Often legumes such as chickpeas (*nut*) and mung beans (*mash*) are mixed with the rice for extra protein. Pilafs are also made from other grains including millet, barley, and sorgo. All of the Central Asian peoples enjoy tasty flatbreads, dumplings, and pies made with wheat-flour dough. *Manty* (large steamed dumplings filled with meat or vegetables), *chuch-vara* (small boiled dumplings), and *samsa* (baked or fried pies filled with meat or vegetables) are encountered throughout the region. Kazakhstan is also known for its *beliashi* (open-faced pies fried in a skillet). Central Asian flatbreads are baked in a *tandyr*, a clay oven similar to the Indian tandoor. *Non*, a large, flat round bread pricked in a decorative pattern with a special instrument, is the most popular. These round breads were originally baked to mimic the shape of the sun. They are eaten alone or used as a plate to hold meat or vegetable stews.

SEASONINGS

Although different regions favor different spices and seasonings, certain flavors characterize Central Asian cuisine as a whole. Onion is used abundantly, as is the fat of the fat-tailed sheep, which lends intense flavor to meat and vegetable dishes. Hot red pepper and black pepper add heat to a wide variety of dishes. *Zira* (cumin), sesame seed, nigella, basil, dill, cilantro, parsley, and mint are all used to enliven foods from soups to salads to pilafs. Cinnamon and saffron are used less widely. Garlic adds intensity to many dishes, while dried barberries contribute a sour tang.

BEVERAGES

Tea, either black or green, is the most popular beverage of Central Asia; the preference for one type over the other depends on the locale. Kazakhs tend to drink more black tea, while the Kyrgyz enjoy green tea served with milk or cream and slightly salted. In Uzbekistan, black tea is drunk more often than green. Black tea, often in traditional pressed-brick form rather than loose-leaf, is boiled with milk and served as a rich beverage. Central Asians drink tea from

Cumin-Spiced Kebabs with Yoghurt and Mint Sauce

Kebabs, yoghurt sauces, and flatbreads (see the article on Afghan cuisine for a recipe) are enjoyed from India to the Middle East, and are especially common in Central Asia. With ingredients that are easy to find, they form the core of many menus and are served together as a delicious meal that can be put together at any time of year. These cumin-spiced kebabs can be cooked on the barbecue or in the oven using the broiler setting. If you're using bamboo skewers, make sure to soak them for about one hour to avoid burning them while cooking.

Ingredients

2 pounds (900 g) boneless leg of lamb, stewing lamb, or lamb chops, cut into 1-inch (2.5 cm) cubes

Spice Mix

1 teaspoon black peppercorns
1 tablespoon (6 g) cumin seeds
½ teaspoon cayenne pepper
1 teaspoon salt

Yoghurt and Mint Sauce

1½ tablespoons (21 g) minced garlic (3 or 4 cloves)
1 cup (40 g) packed fresh mint leaves, finely chopped
1½ cups (340 ml) plain yoghurt
½ teaspoon salt
½ teaspoon black peppercorns, chopped, crushed, or coarsely ground

Preparation

1. Thread the metal or soaked bamboo skewers with the lamb cubes, leaving some room at the top and bottom for easier handling of the skewers.

2. Grind the peppercorns and cumin seeds together with a mortar and pestle or in a spice grinder, and add the cayenne pepper and salt to taste.

3. Dust the lamb with the spice mix, pressing it lightly to ensure that the spices adhere.

4. Cook on a hot barbecue or under a broiler until browned.

5. To make the sauce, combine the garlic and mint with the yoghurt. Season to taste with salt, pepper, and optional spices. Serve with flatbread or grilled meat.

Source: Inspired by recipes from Jeffrey Alford and Naomi Duguid's *Flatbread: A Baker's Atlas.*

a *pialy*, a bowl-like cup without a handle, and serve it as a ritual part of their hospitality. Other beverages include the aforementioned *koumiss* and *ayran* as well as a variety of refreshing fruit drinks with sugar (*sherbet*).

FRUITS AND VEGETABLES

Kazakhstan is the birthplace of the apple (the name of the capital city of Almaty means "father of apples"), and Uzbekistan and Tajikistan produce exceptionally sweet melons. Other fruits include apricots, peaches, cherries, quince, persimmons, and pomegranates; Central Asian raisins and dried apricots are among the best in the world. The most frequently encountered vegetables are root crops such as carrots, turnips, radishes, onions, and garlic. Carrots alone come in a surprising variety of shapes and colors and have a rich, sweet flavor. Pumpkins and squash are frequently used in soups and as fillings for dumplings and pies. Typically, vegetables are not served alone but are added to soups or paired with meats or pilafs.

SWEETS

Traditional Central Asian sweets consist of fruits or nuts simmered in a sugar- or honey-based syrup, either served as a compote or allowed to dry and crystallize. Often, fruits are boiled down to make *bekmes*, a concentrated syrup. Other desserts include halvah, made from ground sesame seeds, and dough fried in coils or balls and sweetened with syrup. Although European-style cookies and cakes were introduced under Russian rule, they never displaced the traditional Eastern sweets that still constitute the best ending to a Central Asian meal. Ice cream, however, is extremely popular.

Two centuries of Russian domination did little to change the traditional foodways of the region, and Central Asian cuisine today still reflects a historical reliance on meats and cultured dairy products. The local foods also reveal the influence of centuries of trade, from Chinese noodles to tandoor-baked flatbreads to Persian-style pilafs. Central Asian cuisine is much more diverse now than it was in the past, with vegetables and fruits making up a larger part of the diet. One thing that has remained constant over the centuries, however, is Central Asia's great tradition of hospitality, which is still very much alive in the region's many *chai-khanas* (tea houses) as well as in private homes.

Darra GOLDSTEIN
Williams College

Further Reading

Alford, J., & Duguid, N. (2008). *Flatbreads and flavors: a baker's atlas*. New York: William Morrow.

Brittin, H. C. (2011). *The food and culture around the world handbook*. London: Pearson

Buell, Paul. (2006). Steppe foodways and history. *Asian Medicine*, 2(2), 171–203.

Eden, Carolyn, & Ford, Eleanor. (2016). *Samarkand: Recipes & stories from Central Asia & The Caucasus*. London: Kyle Books.

Khramov, V. K. (2014). *Turkmen dastarkhan*. Ashgabat: Turkmen State Publishing Service.

Kim'iagarov, A. (2010). *Classic Central Asian (Bukharian) Jewish cuisine and customs*. New York: Alpha Translation & Publishing.

Mack, G. R., & Surina, A. (2005). *Food culture in Russia and Central Asia*. Westport, CT: Greenwood Press.

Makhmudov, K. (2013). *Uzbek cuisine* (Boris Ushumirskiy, Trans.). CreateSpace Independent Publishing Platform

Pokhlebkin, V. V. (1978). *Natsional'nye kukhni nashikh narodov* [National cuisines of our peoples]. Moscow, Russia: Pishchevaia promyshlennost.

Pokhlebkin, V. V. (1984). *Russian delight: a cookbook of the Soviet peoples* (Theresa Prout, Trans.). London: MacMillan.

Visson, L. (1999). *The art of Uzbek cooking*. New York: Hippocrene Books.

Afghan Cuisine

Afghan cuisine blends the flavors and ingredients of Central Asia, the Middle East, South Asia, and China. Afghanistan's location at the hub of the Silk Road accounts for the wide range of culinary influences on the country, with dishes and accompaniments ranging from traditional Indian breads to meat kebabs typical of Middle Eastern cuisine.

L ittle is known of Afghanistan's pre-agricultural days. Wheat, barley, and sheep and goat herding spread from the Near East after 5000 BCE. Civilization grew slowly after 2500 BCE, with a major hiatus during a dry period about 1500–500 BCE. Soon after that, the Greeks and Macedonians under Alexander the Great (356–323 BCE) conquered the country with heavy fighting, leaving behind garrisons of soldiers and artisans who brought their Hellenic customs and cuisine, notably grapes and wine. This was followed by an unsettled era that included the conquest by the Arabs in the early 700s CE and the rise of Islamic realms to dominance.

Afghanistan rose to prominence and great wealth during Central Asia's glory period, when the Silk Road and trade with India and China were important. Then the Mongol conquests in the thirteenth century, followed not long after by the violent wars of Tamerlane (Timur, 1336–1405) and Babur (1483–1530) led to progressive decline. During stable periods, however, the country's oases became famous for intensive cultivation of fruit, including pomegranates, melons, peaches, and mulberries, as well as roses, which supplied not only flowers but also rosewater for flavoring foods. Vegetables were few, but included large quantities of carrots, onions, Chinese chives, and other high-country plants. Chickpeas and other legumes became common. For a brief period in the eighteenth century, Afghanistan became the center of the Middle East, under the dynamic reign of Nadir Shah (1698–1747), who conquered a vast realm from northwest India through Iran, but his heirs could not hold onto it.

The nineteenth century saw Afghanistan caught in the center of the Great Game—the competition of the British and Russian empires for control of

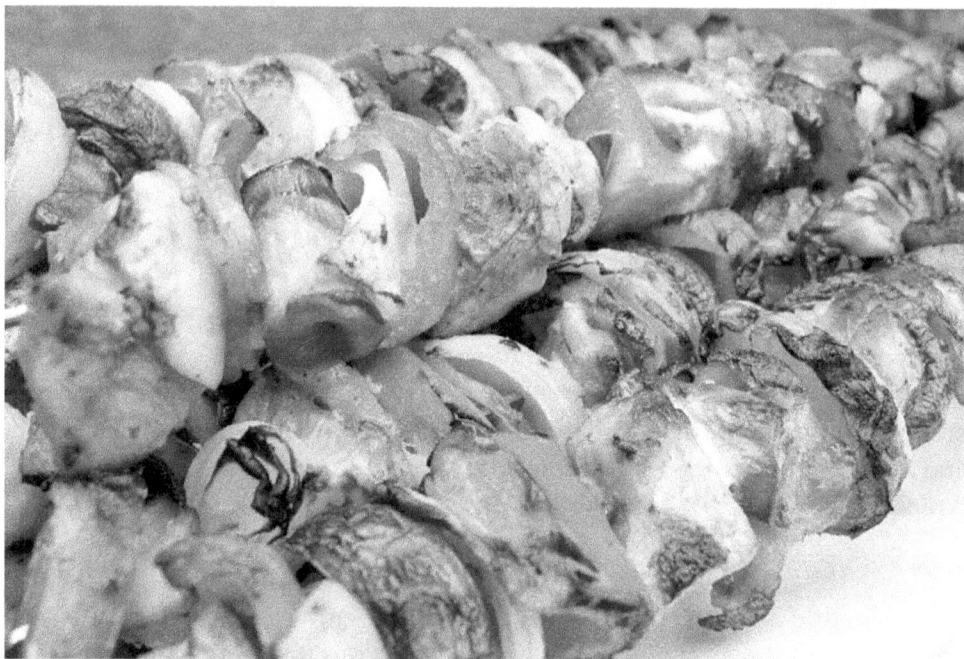

Kebab.

Central Asia. Neither managed to conquer the country, but in the process, potatoes, maize, and chili peppers found their way there from the Americas. The twentieth and twenty-first centuries have brought brief periods of stability between further conflicts and violence.

Characteristics and Ingredients

As the anthropologist Louis Dupree wrote in his survey of Afghanistan, "The Afghan does not live on bread (*nan*) alone but he comes mighty close to it... Throughout much of Afghanistan, the term *nan* refers to food in general. Hot *nan*...is one of the world's great foods" (Dupree 1980, 224). Afghan chef Said Hofioni adds in his book *Afghanistan Cuisine*: "Bread is considered sacred and you shouldn't abuse it or step over it" (Hofiani 2008, 147).

Bread was traditionally made from the hard mountain wheat of the country, which had a special and wonderful flavor. Today, more ordinary flour is usual while other grains, such as barley and maize, are used where wheat does not grow well. Bread is baked in a *tandur*, an oven that can range from a large earthenware jar with thick sides to a vast underground pit. The bread is plastered to the sides, and then carefully removed with a peel board—a difficult operation

Uygur Flatbread

In Afghan cuisine, breads occupy an essential role. This flatbread goes well with the kebabs and yoghurt sauce described in the chapter on Central Asian cuisines. You'll need a baking stone (or quarry tiles) for the best result, but a sturdy baking sheet can also be used. The recipes are inspired by Jeffrey Alford and Naomi Duguid's cookbook *Flatbread: A Baker's Atlas*. Highly recommended by Darra Goldstein, the author of the Central Asia article, this book is packed with recipes from all over the world and includes not just bread, but all kinds of delicious dishes to eat with your breads.

Ingredients
6 cups (720 g) unbleached bread flour, plus more as needed
2¼ teaspoons (7 g) or 1 (¼-ounce) packet of active dry yeast
Sea salt
2½ cups (600 ml) warm water (95°F to 115°F [35°C to 46°C])
Cumin seeds
¼ cup (25 g) finely sliced green onions or chives

Preparation
1. In a large bowl, combine 3 cups (360 g) of the flour with the yeast and a pinch of sea salt. Add the warm water and, using a spoon, stir until the mixture is smooth and stretchy. Continue to add flour until the dough comes away from the sides of the bowl; this could take more or less than 3 more cups (360 g), depending on the moisture content of your flour. Allow to sit for 10 minutes, then knead for 5 to 10 minutes with enough additional flour to prevent sticking.

2. Let the dough rise until it is doubled in size, then punch down, and let it rise again.

3. Arrange a baking stone (or quarry tiles suitable for baking) on the bottom shelf of an oven and preheat it to 500°F (260°C).

4. Divide the dough into 8 pieces, knead each into a neat round, and then roll, pinch, and stretch each one into the largest, flattest shape you can manage. The edges will be thicker, but press the middle until it's thin, stretching the dough as you go. It's okay to have a few stretchy holes. The whole thing will look like a pizza dough ready for its filling. Allow to rise for 10 minutes.

5. Use a fork to prick the entire surface, except for the edges. Sprinkle on the chopped green onions, and then salt and cumin seeds to taste. Press these toppings into the bread, and slide onto the hot stone in the oven.

6. Bake until browned, about 10 minutes.

to manage in a large pit; the bread that falls to the floor is lost. The *nan* is the Persian type: oval, rather thin, leavened, and soft but crusty. Other types of bread include local variants on Indian *chapatis* and *parathas*, as well as cornbread and other local forms.

Breads and noodles are central to meals in Afghanistan. Short-grain rice is used for *bata* (sticky rice), and long-grain rice is the basis for a wide variety of flavorful *pilaus*—rice cooked with meat and spices. A signature dish of Kabul and its region is *qabuli pilau*, made with mutton or lamb, carrots, raisins, spices including black pepper and sometimes cinnamon, cumin, and others, and a lot of *dumba*—the tail fat of the fat-tailed sheep (or, today, rather less oil, and of vegetable sources). Its name, surprisingly, has nothing to do with Kabul; it is probably an Urdu word for "flavorful." The universal snack is kebab—bits of meat on a skewer, usually alternated with some *dumba* to lubricate the often-tough meat. Fried turnovers stuffed with potatoes (*bulani*) or vegetables (*samusa*) are popular appetizers. Spices such as saffron, cumin, mint, cardamom, orange peel, cinnamon, and Chinese chives are part of many dishes. As a general rule, the closer to India, the more the spicing. Raisins and nuts, especially pistachios, almonds, and walnuts (the last largely in eastern mountain valleys), are often-used ingredients as well. Dairy products include yoghurt in various forms, as well as *qurt* (the word is Turkic)—basically dried skim milk, though preparation varies. It is a hard, chewy cake of low-fat milk solids, ideal as a traveling ration for Afghanistan's many nomads, merchants, and traveling workers. Also typical, especially near India, are *dal*—dishes of split peas and beans, with chickpeas and *urd dal* (*Vigna mungo*) being particularly common.

Vegetables are more widely available than meat. Pumpkin is used as the main ingredient for turnovers and soups, and eggplant and spinach figure prominently in many dishes. Lamb is the most popular meat and is used in curries, kebabs, and stews (*korma*). Dumplings are very common, and are often served in a rich sauce; *ashak* or *oshak*, particularly notable, uses tomato sauce and leeks or Chinese chives. Recipes also include ground beef, chicken, and goat. Although spices in these dishes are wide ranging and exotic, Afghan cooking is considered to be somewhat mild compared to other Asian cuisines.

Seasonal fresh fruits such as melons and grapes (Afghanistan is famous for both) are often served at the conclusion of a meal. Sweet treats are considered an extravagance and are not routinely served, but such foods as *firni* (a milky pudding flavored with rose water and pistachios), baklava, and halvah would be among the dessert items for special occasions.

As in most of the world, weddings generally bring out the finest and most elaborate cuisine. Traditionally, a wedding was not merely between two young people; it was an alliance between two tribes, families, or neighborhoods, so everyone entered into the celebration. Also, great feasts were given in the old days, and still are in some cases, by warlords seeking power; fighting men would naturally be attracted, or their loyalty made more firm, by the goodwill generated by such events. Religious festivals such as the *Id* (*Eid*) feast at the end of the fasting month of Ramadan call forth special foods, typically many types of *pilaus* and sweets.

E. N. ANDERSON

University of California, Riverside

Further Reading

Amiri, M. M. (2002). *Classic Afghan cookbook*. Published by the author.

Bourguignon, J. (2006). Jaunt through Asia. *Far Eastern Economic Review, 169*(9), 77.

Dupree, L. (1966). *Kabul gets a supermarket: the birth and growth of an Afghan enterprise*. New York: American Universities Field Staff.

Dupree, L. (1968). *A Kabul supermarket revisited: a successful Afghan entrepreneur views the future*. New York, N.Y.: American Universities Field Staff.

Dupree, L. (1980). *Afghanistan* (2nd Ed.). Princeton, NJ: Princeton University Press.

Eden, Carolyn, & Ford, Eleanor. (2016). *Samarkand: Recipes & stories from Central Asia & The Caucasus*. London: Kyle Books.

Hofioni, S. Z. (2008). *Afghanistan cuisine*. United States: Xlibris.

Lindsay, A., & Lindsay, R. (2009). *Food of the world*. Chandni Chowk, Delhi: Global Media.

Oudenhoven, F. van, & Haider, J. (2015). *With our own hands. A celebration of food and life in the Pamir mountains of Afghanistan and Tajikistan*. Arnhem, Netherlands: Stichting LM Publishers / KIT.

Pant, P., & Mohsin, H. (2005). *Food path cuisine along the Grand Trunk road, from Kabul to Kolkata*. New Delhi: Roli Books.

Parenti, C., & Renella, R. (1987). *A taste of Afghanistan: the cuisine of the crossroads of the world*. Phoenix, AZ: C. Parenti.

Saberi, H. (2004). *Noshe Djan Afghan Food & Cookery*. New York: Marion Boyars.

Saberi, H., Breshna, A., & Zaka, N. (2002). *Afghan food & cookery*. New York: Hippocrene Books.

Safi, N. (2016). *Afghan Food: Healthy Eating*. Authorhouse.

Sekandari, N. (2003). *Afghan cuisine, cooking for life: a collection of Afghan recipes (and other favorites) for the novice Afghan and non-Afghan cook*. Bloomington, IN: 1stBooks.

Sekandari, N. (2010). *Afghan cuisine: a collection of family recipes*. Fremont, CA: Avagana Pub.

Sheen, B. (2011). *Foods of Afghanistan*. Detroit, MI : Gale, Cengage Learning.

Iranian Cuisine

Iranian cuisine reflects the country's history, its geography, and the lifestyle of its people. Composed of locally produced ingredients, the flavors derive from the combinations of these ingredients along with the subtle addition of spices. The result, highly dependent on a cook's technique, is an incredible array of dishes that are popular worldwide and have influenced the cuisines of nearby countries and those as far away as Central Asia.

Iranian cuisine is the product of the skill, creativity, patience, care, and compassion of many generations of cooks—whether mothers, fathers, wives, or husbands preparing food for their families or professional cooks at royal courts and the homes of the affluent. Like all cuisines, the Iranian culinary tradition has also evolved throughout the course of centuries, and it is a reflection of the evolution of indigenous foods as well as adaptations from other cultures.

Because of its relatively large size and diverse climates (from the Persian Gulf in the south to the Caspian Sea in the north), its history of several thousand years, and the many ethnic groups that populate and have populated it, Iran has a rich variety of foods that differ from region to region and sometimes even season to season. The national cuisine of Iran, however, which has spread to and influenced the cuisines of other cultures and countries in South and Central Asia and the Middle East, consists of ethnic and regional foods that have been refined and perfected over the course of many centuries, particularly by the master chefs of the royal courts. To Western tastes, Iranian food seems both exotic and familiar: exotic because the many combinations of vegetables, herbs, spices, and fruits are new; familiar because almost all the ingredients are readily available or commonly used in the West. What characterizes this cuisine is essentially its emphasis on the subtlety of flavors.

Braised Poultry in Walnut and Pomegranate Sauce

Fesenjan

The *fesanjun* sauce should be sweet and sour. Because pomegranate syrup or molasses can vary in sweetness, taste before adding the sugar or lemon juice, and adjust these ingredients accordingly.

Serves 8 to 10

Ingredients
2½ cups (300 g) walnuts, coarsely ground
2 medium onions, grated
¼ cup (60 ml) olive oil
5 tablespoons (80 g) tomato paste
2 tablespoons (30 ml) lemon juice
3 tablespoons (38 g) sugar
½ cup (120 ml) pomegranate syrup or molasses*
½ teaspoon cinnamon
¼ teaspoon ground black pepper
2 teaspoons (12 g) salt
4 pounds (2 kg) boneless, skinless chicken thighs or breasts**
2 tablespoons (30 g) butter

Note
*If pomegranate syrup or molasses is not available, cranberry jelly can be substituted, in which case the sugar should be reduced or eliminated altogether.

** Substitute 5 pounds (2.3 kg) duck for the chicken and increase the simmering time until the duck is tender, adding water, if necessary.

Preparation
1. Lightly brown the walnuts in a heavy dry skillet over low heat, stirring constantly to prevent burning. Transfer to a 5- to 6-quart (4.75 to 5.5 L) saucepot.

2. In the same skillet, sauté the onions lightly in the oil. Remove the onions with a slotted spoon and add them to the walnuts. Set the skillet aside.

3. Add all remaining ingredients except the chicken and butter to the walnut-onion mixture, along with 2½ cups (600 ml) water. Mix well. Simmer over low heat for 10 minutes.

4. Melt the butter in a skillet and brown the chicken; add it to the sauce, cover, and simmer for approximately 1 hour, stirring occasionally to prevent sticking. Serve over plain rice.

Source: M. R. Ghanoonparvar. (2006). *Persian cuisine: Traditional, regional, and modern foods*. Costa Mesa, CA: Mazda Publishers.

Characteristics

Although food is an essential need for human survival, the traditions of food preparation that comprise the cuisine of every tribe, ethnic group, or nation represent that culture, and are indeed regarded as a way of celebrating that culture. Combining various edible ingredients, devising different methods of preparation, and arranging and decorating various dishes for presentation at the table to members of families and guests is an art developed in every culture over many generations that requires not only skill, creativity, and patience, but also care and compassion.

Based on the ingredients used and methods of preparation, Iranian foods are categorized into a dozen or so main groups, some of which are *polo* (rice mixed with other ingredients such as legumes, meats, vegetables, and herbs), *khoresh* (stew-type dishes that are usually served over *chelo*, or plain rice), *kabab* (skewered meats), *ash* (thick pottage-like dishes), *abgusht* (soups), *dolmeh* (stuffed vegetables and grape leaves), *kufteh* (meat and/or rice balls), and *kuku* (vegetable or other soufflé-type dishes). Rice is one of the most important staples in the Iranian diet and is often the main dish. The most popular way of making rice in Iran, which is quite different from that of most other cuisines, results in fluffy, separated grains of rice. For this kind of dish, a high quality, long-grain rice such as Basmati is used, which has a unique flavor and aroma. Traditionally, red meat and poultry are not consumed in the quantities that are customary in the West. Meats are often used to flavor dishes, as are other ingredients. Iranian foods are by no means bland, which is not to say that they are spicy, as is typically associated with Indian and some Mexican cuisines, for example. A typical Iranian meal may consist of a rice dish with a meat sauce; yoghurt; fresh herbs such as mint, basil, and tarragon; and freshly baked bread, of which there are many varieties available on every street corner.

Depending on such factors as the culinary traditions of various ethnic groups in Iran and the country's diverse climates and agricultural products, one could speak of several traditions of cooking in the country. On the whole, however, and especially in more recent centuries, a sizable number of dishes with usually the same ingredients and preparation methods have become common in all parts of the country, although one would find slight regional or personal variations.

Ingredients

With the exception of some spices, almost all agricultural as well as dairy products and meats used in Iran are produced domestically. Up to about a century ago, other than a relatively small percentage of the population who lived in the major cities, the majority of the Iranian people either lived in small villages that provided the agricultural products, or they were migrating nomads who produced dairy products as well as red meats, mainly mutton. Many varieties of vegetables, herbs, grains, fruits, and nuts that are a part of the Iranian diet have been cultivated in the country since ancient times. The most common traditional vegetables and legumes are eggplants, zucchinis, cucumbers, onions, lettuce, spinach, leeks, chickpeas, lentils, mung beans, fava beans, and split peas, while tomatoes and potatoes have been added to this list in recent centuries. In Iran, herbs such as spearmint, basil, dill, coriander, parsley, and fenugreek are considered vegetables and are served either raw or in certain prepared dishes. Among the grains, wheat and rice are the most common. Bread is served with every meal, and although barley was also used in the past for making bread, especially in villages, wheat remains the predominant grain for making a variety of flatbreads. Rice, which was mainly served in affluent families until a couple of centuries ago, has now become a part of virtually every Iranian's diet and is the main staple—served either as plain rice, accompanied by stew-like dishes of mutton or chicken and vegetables and fruits, or mixed with other ingredients and served as a complete meal. In addition to the vegetables and herbs that enhance the taste and subtle aroma of rice, stews, soups, and other categories of Iranian cuisine, the most common spices that are used include turmeric, salt, black pepper, cinnamon, oregano, and of course Iranian saffron, the most expensive spice in the world. A cook's skill and talent are usually judged not only by how he or she has prepared the rice, but also—just as importantly—by how he or she has combined the ingredients and seasoned the sauce that is served with it. A typical stew-type topping that is served with fluffy rice is, for instance, *fesenjan,* which is a sweet and sour dish consisting of braised poultry, walnuts, onions, and pomegranate molasses. Another popular dish served with rice is called *qormeh sabzi,* which is made with cubes of mutton, onions, scallions, parsley, dried whole limes, and fenugreek (which provides the main flavor), and is seasoned with salt, pepper, and turmeric.

Among dairy products, the most common is yoghurt, which is often served as a side dish with lunch and dinner, sometimes mixed with vegetables such as cucumbers or cooked spinach. The traditional cheeses in Iran are goat feta and a crumbled goat cheese. Butter, ghee, and whey are also important in Iranian cuisine. Butter has been traditionally and mainly used in making confections, ghee has been the main oil used in rice dishes as well as for frying, and whey has been served with a variety of thick soups and eggplant dishes. In the past, because of the lack of refrigeration, with the exception of those who lived near the Caspian Sea and the Persian Gulf, seafood was not part of the everyday diet in Iran. That being said, however, fried smoked fish served with herbs and cooked with rice is the traditional meal for the Iranian New Year, which is celebrated on the first day of spring.

Finally, an important aspect of Iranian cuisine is the presentation of the dishes. Rice is usually decorated with a layer of saffron-flavored grains of rice, and various stews and soups are topped with designed patterns made with yoghurt or whey, caramelized sliced onions, nuts, cinnamon, and so on.

M. R. GHANOONPARVAR
University of Texas at Austin

Further Reading

Batmanglij, N. (1992). *The new food of life: A book of ancient Persian and modern Iranian cooking and ceremonies*. Washington, DC: Mage Publishers.

Bundy, A., & Linder, L. (2012). *Pomegranates and roses: My Persian family recipes*. London: Simon & Schuster.

Chehabi, H. E. (2003). The westernization of Iranian culinary culture. *Iranian Studies*, 2003, 43–61.

Dana-Haeri, J. (2014). *From a Persian kitchen: Fresh discoveries in Iranian cooking*. New York: I.B. Tauris.

Ghanoonparvar, M. R. (2016). *Dining at the Safavid court*. Costa Mesa, CA: Mazda Publishers.

Ghanoonparvar, M. R. (2006). *Persian cuisine: Traditional, regional, and modern foods*. Costa Mesa, CA: Mazda Publishers.

Hekmat, F. (1961). *The art of Persian cooking*. Garden City, NY: Hippocrene Books.

Karizaki, Vahid Mohammadpour. (2017). Ethnic and traditional Iranian breads: different types, and historical and cultural aspects. *Journal of Ethnic Foods*, 4(1), 8–14.

Karizaki, Vahid Mohammadpour. (2016). Ethnic and traditional Iranian rice-based foods. *Journal of Ethnic Foods*, 3(2), 124–134.

Karizaki, Vahid Mohammadpour. (2017). Iranian dates and ethnic date-based products. *JEF Journal of Ethnic Foods*, 4(3), 204–209.

Mazda, M. (1980). *In a Persian kitchen: Favorite recipes from the Near East*. Rutland, VT: Tuttle Publishing.

Malouf, G., Malouf, L., Bayat, E. K., & Roper, M. (2012). *Saraban: A chef's journey through Persia*. Richmond: Hardie Grant Books.

Parvaneh Seyed Almasi. (2013). The impact of traditional medicine on Iranian cuisine ingredients. *Asian Journal of Natural and Applied Sciences*, 2(3), 90–97.

Ramazani, N. (1982). *Persian cooking. A table of exotic delights*. Charlottesville, VA: University Press of Virginia. 1982.

Sedghi, H. (2007). *Feast of flavours from the Iranian kitchen: a step-by-step culinary adventure*. Singapore: Marshall Cavendish Cuisine.

Shaida, M. (2002). *The legendary cuisine of Persia*. New York: Interlink Books.

Simmons, S. (2002). *A treasury of Persian cuisine*. East Sussex: The Book Guild.

Shafia, L. (2013). *The new persian kitchen*. New York: Ten Speed Press.

Shaida, M. (2017). *The legendary cuisine of Persia*. Northampton, MA: Interlink Books.

Vladica, E. (2010). Tastes of Persian & Armenian cuisine: selections of popular and easy recipes. Castle Hill, Australia: E. Vladica.

Iraqi Cuisine

Developed over five thousand years of history, the cuisine of Iraq ranges from rustic to refined and includes lamb stews, stuffed foods, pastries, and flatbread baked in clay ovens. The spice trade and influences from the New World enhanced the flavors of traditional dishes, while the development of the sugar industry gave rise to the creation of countless syrupy desserts.

Iraq's cuisine reflects its topographical and ethnic diversity. Located in the western corner of Asia, Iraq was first named Mesopotamia (land between two rivers), as both the Tigris and Euphrates rivers run through it. The north is partially mountainous, and mostly inhabited by the Kurds and other ethnic minorities. The rest of the country is made up of a fertile plain populated mostly by Arabs, and a western desert inhabited by nomadic Bedouins.

Iraqis enjoy a refined cuisine with roots in over five thousand years of documented history from Mesopotamian times, through the golden medieval era when Baghdad ruled the Arabo-Islamic world, on to the present. The myriad variety of dishes range from stews of mutton and vegetables served with rice and bread, to dishes of fish and elaborate stuffed and rolled meats, vegetables, and pastries. For Iraqis, whose lives have been disrupted by wars and political strife, this brilliant culinary heritage is a source of pride and solace.

Foodstuffs and Dishes

The diversity of the land of Iraq and its people has inevitably influenced its cuisine, which is vast and varied, albeit more defined by topography than ethnicity or religion. The northern region is where the wheat-based dishes abound, such as those cooked with bulgur (cracked wheat). With its winter and spring rains, this region's lush pastures are not only more conducive to growing wheat but also to the production of delicious sheep and goat yoghurt and cheeses. Hence, more dishes here are cooked with yoghurt. On the other hand, Iraqis in the middle and southern regions, dependent on the two rivers for irrigation, are more barley and rice-eaters. Barley is more tolerant of heat and salinity, and rice thrives in the paddies of the southern marshlands, or *al-Ahwar*, where the aromatic rice *timman ambar* (ambergris rice) grows.

The spiciest dishes are relished in the southern city of Basra, which has a long trade history with India, from which the best spices were imported. The spice blend generally used in Iraq is called *baharat*, which is a brownish spice mix of many ingredients including cardamom, cinnamon, ginger, cloves, and allspice. The other spice mix is called *bahar asfar*, which is a yellow spice blend similar to curry powder. The city's spiciness is boosted by a delicately tangy dried lime called *noomi Basra*, which, though named after the city, is in fact imported from Oman.

Many varieties of fruit trees grow in the entire region, the most important of which is the date palm, acclaimed as the national tree of the land. To the ancient inhabitants of Iraq, it was their tree of life. Hundreds of date varieties are grown, all in the warmer central and southern regions. Besides eating fresh and dried dates as fruit, Iraqis also make date syrup, or *dibis*. In the northern region, honey is the counterpart to *dibis*, due to the area's weather and resources.

Mutton is preferred over other meats, particularly for stews that require chunks on the bone. It is not cheap, however, and the quantity consumed depends on one's means. Goat meat is mostly eaten in the mountainous region, and beef is generally ground. Pork is hard to find since the majority of Iraqis are Muslims, and camel meat is mostly confined to the desert area. Domestic chicken is generally tough, and it is always boiled before doing anything else with it. Before the economic sanctions in the 1990s and the ensuing wars, substantial amounts of frozen chicken used to be imported. As for fish, the major sources are the Tigris and Euphrates. It is more relished in the central and southern regions than in the north. The southern port city of Basra, with access to the Gulf, is where shrimp and sea fish are mostly consumed. The southern marsh people of al-Ahwar still salt and dry fish like their ancient ancestors used to do. Vegetables are seasonal and consumed by all indiscriminately. Eggplant and zucchini are ubiquitous, but the most beloved of all is okra. Lentils, mung beans, and other dried beans are handy when fresh vegetables in winter are not as abundant and varied as they are in summertime.

Cooking Techniques

Stews served with rice or bulgur are the daily staple of all Iraqis. Chunks of lamb on the bone are simmered in tomato-based broth along with a seasonal vegetable. The rice is often served plain, but can be prepared in a variety of ways, depending on occasion and affordability. For special events, it may be attractively colored—yellow with turmeric, saffron for those who can afford it, or red with tomato sauce—and garnished with fried raisins and sliced almonds.

Iraqi cuisine is also distinguished by an impressive array of elaborate dishes: an assortment of vegetables are cored and stuffed with a flavorful and aromatic mix of rice and ground meat to make a pot of juicy simmered *dolma*. Dough made of bulgur, boiled rice, or boiled potatoes, is stuffed with a spicy mix of ground meat cooked with onion, to make variously shaped *kubba*, and fried in vegetable oil. For big gatherings, the dish to offer is *qoozi*, a whole lamb stuffed with rice, nuts, and raisins and then baked to succulence. A chicken may be prepared similarly, but it is additionally stuffed underneath its entire skin. The simple and yet unique fish dish of *masgoof* is the specialty of fishermen along the banks of the Tigris river in Baghdad. Fish, sliced open, are hung from the back on forked stakes and left to bake slowly around an open campfire. Since ancient times, Iraqis have been cooking this remarkable repertoire of dishes—and many others.

The Historical Scene

Cooking with water is recognized as an advanced stage in human history. Relatively recent archaeological findings have confirmed that this cooking technique had been perfected in ancient Iraq a few millennia ago. The most tangible evidence is found in three 1700 BCE cuneiform clay tablets excavated in Babylon, seventy miles south of present-day Baghdad. The tablets contain twenty-four recipes for stew dishes cooked with meat and vegetables, enhanced with sheep-tail fat, and seasoned with leeks, onion, garlic, spices, and herbs like cassia, cumin, coriander, mint, and dill. Included are several recipes that deal with stuffed bird pies, which are by far the first documented examples of stuffed dishes. Wheat-based flatbread was baked in clay ovens, called *tinuru* back then. Similar clay ovens are common to this day, and they are called by the same name.

The medieval era marked the zenith of the region's prosperity, when Baghdad was founded by the Abbasid caliphate in 762 CE. Baghdad soon became a thriving trade center strategically located at the crossroads of the Eastern and Western cultures of Persia, Greece, and Rome. Baghdadi cuisine was renowned for its remarkable diversity and sophistication. Both professional cooks and lovers of food from all walks of life experimented with dishes and wrote about it. The several extant cookbooks from that period represent only the tip of the iceberg of what was written at the time. From them we learn that stew was the

White Beans and Beet Salad

Zalatat Fasulya Yabsa wa Shuwandar

This is typically a winter salad in Iraq. Because tomatoes are scarce and expensive during this season, beets are usually substituted to add color and flavor to salads. You can easily boil the white beans and the beets separately beforehand so that you can put the salad together in no time. Alternatively, you may use canned white beans, but remember to rinse and drain the beans before adding them to the salad. Feel free to adjust seasonings to suit your taste.

Serves 4

Ingredients
2 cups (480 ml) cooked white beans
2 medium beets (about 1 pound), boiled, peeled, and cut into small cubes
½ medium onion, sliced very thinly crosswise
2 tablespoons (30 ml) olive oil
Juice of half a lemon or 2 tablespoons (30 ml) vinegar
¼ teaspoon salt
¼ teaspoon ground black pepper
¼ teaspoon chili pepper
½ teaspoon sugar
Chopped parsley, for garnish

Preparation
In a large serving bowl, combine all the ingredients except for the parsley and mix well. Garnish with the chopped parsley and serve.

Source: Nawal Nasrallah

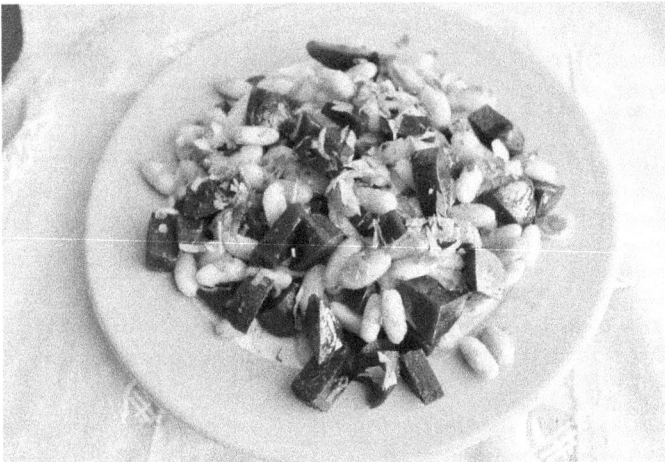

mainstay even then, served with flatbreads baked in clay ovens. Stuffed dishes were a source of pride and an occasion for showmanship on the part of the cooks. The rise of the sugar industry during this period gave rise to the creation of countless syrupy desserts and *halva*, which still characterize the Iraqi sweets scene of today.

Later, ingredients from the New World, like tomatoes, changed the Iraqi way of cooking stews. Tomatoes gradually replaced most of the thickening, souring, and coloring agents used in the preparation of stews, such as nuts, sour juice of fruits and vegetables, saffron, and pomegranate juice. Only a few tomato-less dishes of stew remain today, such as *summaqiyya* (soured and colored with sumac berries) of the northern city of Mosul and *rummaniyya*, now called *fasanjun* (soured with pomegranate and thickened with walnut) south of Baghdad. In addition, sheep-tail fat, deemed a delicacy until recently, is sparingly used these days due to health considerations.

Since the early 1990s, Iraq has been going through harsh political conditions with significant economic consequences. The destruction of infrastructure and diminishing oil revenues have kept the majority of Iraqis under oppressive economic conditions. But history tells us that cuisines endure with their peoples, and Iraqis are no different, both in their homeland and in the diaspora. A case in point is the destruction of whole date palm orchards in the past three decades due to conflicts or neglect, which has decimated a crop with importance for the country and its culture. Yet re-planting programs and plans for the appearance of the palm tree in new designs of the Iraqi flag are positive signs for the culture and its cuisine.

Nawal NASRALLAH

Independent scholar, USA

Further Reading

Bottéro, J. (2004). *The Oldest Cuisine in the World: Cooking in Mesopotamia*. (T. L. Fagan, Trans.). Chicago, IL: University of Chicago Press.

Miller, H.D. (2007). The pleasures of consumption: The birth of Medieval Islamic cuisine. In Paul Freedman (Ed.), *Food: The history of taste* (pp. 135–161). Berkeley, CA: University of California Press.

Nasrallah, N. (2008). The Iraqi cookie, *kleicha*, and the search for identity. *Repast*, 24 (4), 4–7. Retrieved June 7, 2016, from http://www.iraqicookbook.com/yahoo_site_admin/assets/docs/2008_Fall.21212755.pdf

Nasrallah, N. (2013). *Delights from the Garden of Eden: A cookbook and history of the Iraqi cuisine*. Sheffield, UK: Equinox Publishing.

Turkish Cuisine

Turkish cuisine is known the world over for its rich, intricate flavors. Benefitting both from its location along the Silk Road and from the extent of fertile lands that have given it a self-sufficiency few other countries enjoy, Turkish cuisine developed into a plethora of dishes enjoyed today both at home and at restaurants.

Turkey, the unique Muslim Republic with a democratic and secular regime, located in the eastern Mediterranean where it bridges Europe and Asia, has always been a bridge between European and Middle Eastern cultures with its historic and contemporary customs and traditional cuisine.

The richness and diversity of Turkish cuisine is a result of the Ottoman empire (453–1922), which reigned for centuries over a varied geography and landscape combining characteristics of Europe, Africa, and Asia, and which interacted with different cultures throughout the centuries. Turkish cuisine thus has many specialties and variations, and it is understandable that people from Greece or Lebanon would claim that *moussaka*, for instance, is a Greek or Lebanese dish.

Meals at Home and in Restaurants

Turkish cuisine generally consists of soups; salads; sauced dishes prepared with cereals, vegetables, and meat; pastries with meat and vegetable fillings; cold vegetable dishes cooked in olive oil; and flour- and semolina-based desserts.

A typical Turkish breakfast consists of white cheese, fresh tomatoes, black or green olives or both, honey and jam, boiled eggs, fresh bread from the bakery, and tea. New healthy eating habits imported from Europe and the United States, such as consuming cereals and fruits, are welcomed by Turkish families. Consumption of meat products such as ham or sausage, however, is still not popular.

107

Families and working people who lack the time to get together tend to skip lunch. In restaurants, however, the lunch served includes soup, seasoned lamb or chicken with vegetables, a rice- or bulgur- (cracked and boiled wheat) pilaf dish, and salad. Milk desserts are preferred for lunch.

Most Turkish dinners start with appetizers called *meze*. *Meze* are a category of food consumed in small quantities at the start of a meal and traditionally intended to accompany alcoholic drinks, especially raki, an anise-flavored liqueur. White-bean salad, smoked eggplant puree, green salads, pickles, feta cheese, fresh vegetables drenched in yoghurt sauce and garlic, pastrami (dried tenderloin or sirloin), *tarama* (fish puree), humus (chickpea puree), and fava (broad-bean puree) are served as *mezes*. The main course that follows is grilled or fried fish or meat with fried tomatoes, green pepper, and sautéed potatoes. Fruits and desserts are served before enjoying Turkish coffee.

Ingredients

The intricate flavors of Turkish cuisine depend on local food products and fresh meat and vegetables. Traditionally, the fertile lands of the country, which stretch for a thousand miles from east to west, have provided the gamut of foods that Turks still enjoy today.

VEGETABLES

Vegetables are consumed in large quantities and generally are not boiled in water or used as garniture. It is customary to cook vegetables with meat, onions, tomatoes, or tomato paste. Vegetables are also cooked in olive oil. A specialty of Turkish cuisine is the *zeytinyagli* or olive-oil course. Oil is important in Turkish cuisine. Vegetables, such as root celery, green string beans, artichokes, leeks, eggplants, or zucchini can be cooked in olive oil and served at room temperature. Vegetables such as peppers, eggplants, carrots, or zucchinis can also be fried and served with a tomato-garlic or yoghurt-garlic sauce.

Onion and tomatoes are the main ingredients of almost all dishes. Chopped onions fried in oil and fresh tomatoes (or tomato paste) are added to dishes and are also chopped into most salads.

Dolma is the term for stuffed vegetables. There are two kinds of *dolma*: those filled with ground meat and eaten with a yoghurt sauce, and those with seasoned rice mix and cooked in olive oil. The former is a frequent main-course dish. Any vegetable that can be filled with or wrapped around these mixes can be used to prepare *dolma*: zucchini, pepper, tomato, cabbage, grape leaf, and eggplant are examples of such vegetables. Eggplant (or aubergine) has a special place in Turkish cuisine.

MEAT

Meat is very important in Turkish cuisine, and sheep, lamb, beef, and veal are often served, along with vegetables, in dishes made at home. The real taste and flavor of meat, however, can be best appreciated by tasting kebabs at restaurants. Kebab is widespread in many Mid-Eastern countries, but is originally Turkish. *Shish* kebab is grilled cubes of skewered lamb or veal. *Döner* kebab is made by stacking layers of ground meat and sliced leg of lamb on a large upright skewer, which is slowly rotated in front of a vertical charcoal fire. As the outer layer of the meat is roasted, thin slices can be cut and served with rice pilaf. Southern and southeastern cities of Turkey are famous for the variety of their kebabs.

PILAF, BREADS, AND PASTRIES

Pilaf, another specialty of Turkish cuisine, is popular both domestically and abroad. The most common types are cracked-wheat pilaf and rice pilaf. Pilaf is made of rice boiled in beef stock with cubed onions and tomatoes and green peppers sautéed in butter, and it is usually served with vegetable and meat dishes.

Accompanying the main dishes is a variety of bread made of wheat and corn flour. Pita, a flatbread with various toppings, *simit*, ring bread with sesame seed, and *manti* (Turkish ravioli) are some examples of breads and pastries. But the true specialty is the *börek*, a special pastry of thin sheets of homemade dough (*yufka*). The pastry sheets are layered or folded into various shapes after being filled with cheese, vegetable, meat, or other mixes, and then are baked or fried.

SPICES AND SEASONINGS

Situated at the crossroads of Europe and Asia, Turkey welcomed traders on the camel caravans that plied the Silk Road, carrying spices from the East. Many of these spices are still used in Turkish cooking, the most common being red pepper, cinnamon, thyme, and cumin. Widely used seasonings are dill, mint, parsley, and garlic. Fresh or dried mint is also consumed.

YOGHURT, DESSERTS, AND BEVERAGES

Yoghurt, invented by herders of Central Asia, is a contribution of Turkish cuisine to the world, and remains a popular food and a staple in the Turkish diet. Turkish chefs can cite at least a hundred recipes in which yoghurt is used as an ingredient or a sauce. *Ayran*, a widely consumed national non-alcoholic drink, is a diluted and salted sour yoghurt, served with meals or with snacks.

Desserts are another specialty of Turkish cuisine, the best-known being Turkish delight (*lokum*) and baklava. *Lokum* is a jelly sweet often mixed with walnuts or pistachios, cut into cubes, and rolled in powdered sugar. Baklava is the paper-thin pastry sheets that are brushed with butter and folded, layered, or rolled after being filled with ground pistachios, walnuts or heavy cream, baked, then soaked with a thick syrup.

Traditional drinks in Turkey include strong Turkish coffee, preferred after meals, and Turkish tea (*cay*), with its deep red color and unique taste.

Turkish Coffee

In the preparation of Turkish coffee, sugar is added during the brewing process, not after, and it is served unfiltered in small cups.

Ingredients

1 cup (240 ml) cold water
Sugar (optional)
1 tablespoon (6 g) extra finely ground
   coffee (should be powder consistency)

⅛ teaspoon ground cardamom, or
   1 cardamom pod

Preparation

1. Bring the water and sugar to taste, if desired, to a boil in an *ibrik*, a small coffeepot, or a small saucepan.

2. Remove from the heat and stir in the coffee and cardamom.

3. Return the saucepan to the heat and allow it to come to a boil. Remove from heat when the coffee foams.

4. Again, return to the heat, allowing it to foam, and remove from the heat.

5. Pour the coffee into 2 small demitasse cups and allow it to sit for a few minutes so the grounds settle to the bottom of the cups. The cardamom pod can be served with the coffee for added flavor.

Source: Adapted from the website The Spruce (https://www.thespruce.com/turkish-coffee-recipe-2355497)

Turkish Tea

Turkish tea is traditionally brewed using a two-storied teapot (*çaydanlık*), where the bottom part is used to boil the water, while the top holds the brewed tea. It is served in special small, thin-walled glasses, first filling them to a quarter, one-third, or half of the glass with the brewed tea (depending on the strength of the tea), and then topping them off with hot water.

▶▶

Muhallebi, made with milk, sugar, and rice flour, is a traditional dessert in Turkish cuisine, as is *halvah,* made by pan-sautéing semolina and pine nuts in butter before adding sugar, milk, or water and briefly cooking until these are absorbed.

Turkish traditional drinks include strong Turkish coffee, preferred after meals, and Turkish tea, with its deep red color and unique taste. *Cay,* Turkish tea, is brewed over boiling water; it is served in special small, thin-walled glasses.

Ingredients
7 cups (1.7 L) water
5 tablespoons (30 g) black tea leaves

Traditional preparation using a two-storied *çaydanlık*
1. Fill the bottom kettle with water and bring to boil over high heat on your stove top.
2. Place the tea leaves into the upper kettle and stack it on top of the bottom one.
3. Once the water in the bottom kettle boils, pour half into the upper kettle to brew the tea.
4. Reduce the heat to medium and let the tea brew for 15 to 20 minutes in the upper kettle over the steam coming from the bottom kettle.
5. Pour some of the brewed tea into a Turkish tea glass up to the waist (the narrowest part of the tea glass) and then dilute it with hot water from the bottom kettle.

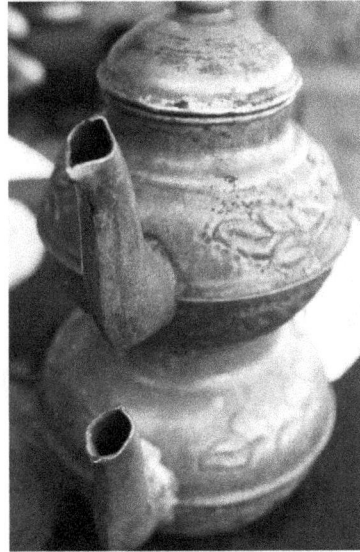
A two-storied Turkish teapot.

Preparation without a Turkish teapot
1. Fill two pots with water: a small pot for a very strong tea brew and a larger pot or kettle for additional boiled water.
2. Bring the smaller pot of water to a boil. Add 1 teaspoon of tea for each glass you will serve and allow the mixture to brew for about 10 minutes.
3. In the meantime, boil additional water in the larger pot or kettle.
4. Pour some of the brewed tea into a Turkish tea glass up to the waist (the narrowest part of the tea glass) and then dilute it with hot water.
5. Serve with sugar, if desired, and Turkish delight (optional, but highly recommended)

Sources: Adjusted from *Turkish Coffee and Tea World* (https://www.turkishcoffeeworld.com/Tea-Pots-s/158.htm) and *Give Recipe* (https://www.giverecipe.com/turkish-tea).

Among alcoholic drinks, raki is usually mixed with water at the table; in everyday language, it is called lion's milk. *Sherefe* (cheers) is a common toast.

Cuisine and Lifestyle

Proud of their cuisine and the richness of its flavors, eating is taken seriously by Turkish people. It is inconceivable for family members to eat alone or eat and run while others are at home. The concept of having a potluck meal at someone's house is also entirely foreign to the Turks. Despite the increasing presence of frozen and canned foods and fast-food chains in the big cities, Turkish cuisine is resisting the new habits of eating, both in domestic settings and in restaurants.

Emel YILMAZ

Co-author of *Turkish Culinary Art: A Journey through Turkish Cuisine*

Further Reading

Akin, E. (2015). *Essential Turkish cuisine*. New York: Stewart, Tabori & Chang.

Arsian, A. B., et al. (2008). *Turkish cuisine*. Ankara: Ministry of Culture and Tourism.

Basan, G. (1997). *Classic Turkish cooking*. New York: St. Martin's Press.

Baysal, A. (1993). *Samples from Turkish cuisine*. Ankara, Turkey: Historical Society.

Bulut, G. B.; Gezgin, N.; & Yilmaz, E. (2014). *Turkish culinary art: A journey through Turkish cuisine*. New York: Blue Dome Press.

Eren, N. (1969). *The art of Turkish cooking, or delectable delights of Topkapi*. Garden City, NY: Doubleday.

Foodstuffs

Rice and Rice Agriculture

Asia is the world's leader in rice production and consumption. Originating and first cultivated in Asia, it is still the dominant crop for millions of people. Thriving in standing water, rice is uniquely adapted to areas with heavy flooding, but also depends on human irrigation. Over time, various types of rice and rice cultivation have developed, with a recent focus on improving rice yield to keep up with population growth.

Rice is Asia's most important food crop, and Asian rice production and consumption account for over 90 percent of the world total. About two-thirds of Asian caloric consumption comes from cereals: about 40 percent of that comes from rice, while 15 percent more is from wheat. Rice and wheat are also the major prestige grains. In areas where rice is the dominant crop, it is almost always symbolic of food and well-being in general. In Japan, the word *gohan* means both rice and meal, the same is true for the Chinese word *fàn* 饭; major deities are associated with rice, and national festivals mark the times of planting, transplanting, and harvest. In southern and eastern India, no meal would be considered complete without rice, even if it also included bread made of some other grain. All over India, a paste of crushed cooked rice and turmeric is the quintessential material for making a *tilak*—the mark made on one's forehead in ceremonies seeking a good beginning, such as weddings.

Rice itself is, however, generally not deified, just as bread is not in the West. Although local deities associated with rice or rice fields are widely reported, the ceremonies associated with them are better understood as ways to take recognized oaths regarding farming arrangements than worship as such.

Rice yield has commonly been used to assess land, and taxes have been levied in rice. Maintaining stable rice prices has been a major concern of government policy for virtually all of recorded history. In recent decades, the improvement of rice production has been a major focus of international development agencies and governments throughout Asia.

115

Origins and Ecology

Rice is unique among the major cereal crops in its ability to grow in standing water. It is therefore uniquely adapted to the periodic heavy flooding that often accompanies Asian monsoons.

Worldwide, there are two domesticated species—*Oryza sativa* and *O. glabberima*—and about twenty-six wild species. *O. sativa* evolved in Asia and is divided into two subspecies: *indica*, which is more prominent in South Asia, and *japonica*, which dominates in East Asia. Both subspecies are now distributed worldwide. *O. glabberima* is indigenous to West Africa and is still localized there. Both domestic species appear to have the same wild ancestor, commonly thought to be *O. rufipogon*, an inhabitant of ponds and flooded ditches.

The main differences between the *indica* and *japonica* subspecies is that the former has a taller growth habit and produces long, thin grains that are separate when cooked. With *japonica*, the grains are shorter and wider, tending to be stickier when cooked, and the plants are shorter stemmed. There is, however, much variation within both groups. The differences involve taste and texture, yield, whether the rice is "floating" or not, the length of time to maturity, and whether the growth cycle is photoperiod-sensitive or not. "Floating" means that the stems tend to lengthen as water depth increases, preventing the plant from drowning in deep water (some floating rice varieties can grow to heights of several meters). Photoperiod sensitivity is the tendency for the time of maturation to be controlled by the length of the day.

It is most likely that *O. sativa* was domesticated from its wild ancestor at several places and at several times. The most likely zone of domestication extends from the upper Ganges and Brahmaputra valleys, across northern Burma and Thailand, and across southern China. It seems probable that *indica-japonica* differentiation occurred in different niches in the eastern Himalayas and into mountainous Southeast Asia, with *japonica* varieties emerging in lowlands and *indica* in uplands. Such differentiation is found in the area today, and the indigenous *aus* and *aman* varieties that are commonly grown as a first and following crop in Bangladesh appear in many characteristics to be midway between the two subspecies.

The earliest evidence of domestication appears to be from China, where carbonized *japonica* grains dating from about 7000 BCE have been found mixed with *O. rufipogon* in the Hemedu site in the lower Yangtze (Chang) River valley. In South Asia, the earliest evidence is from Lothal and Rangpur in Gujarat, dating from 4300 and 4000 BCE, respectively. From Southeast Asia, the oldest evidence comes from Non Nok Tha in Thailand, dating from 5500 BCE. From its origin points, rice has steadily spread north and south through the wetter areas of monsoon Asia, mainly replacing taro-based cultivation systems, such as survive in Papua New Guinea.

Rice and wheat are complementary rather than competitive. Wheat does better in cooler weather, and some wheats have a chilling or freezing requirement before they will form grain, while frost inhibits or kills rice. Rice is, therefore, generally a tropical- and temperate-climate crop, while wheat is a temperate- and cold-climate crop. In areas where both can grow, rice is consistently a summer crop and wheat a winter crop.

Rice is grown in four major ways: in shifting swiddens, on rain-fed dryland like other cereals, in rain-fed flooded fields, and in irrigated flooded fields. Since archaeological evidence of rice consists mainly of carbonized grains or grain-impressions on pottery, it is not known whether rice was originally domesticated as a dryland or wetland crop. While rice yields well without flooding, provided the soil remains moist, under such conditions it is less resistant to weeds than other cereals. Flooding controls weeds and provides an environment in which certain waterweeds (notably Azolla), blue-green algae, and bacteria supply the necessary nitrogen on a sustained basis. Over recent history, flooded cultivation has been consistently more important, and this importance continues to increase.

Different modes of cultivation dominate in different regions. In South Asia, rice cultivation depends entirely on irrigation in Pakistan and from a third to a half on irrigation in India. Although India still has a few pockets of shifting cultivation and some dryland farming along the edges of the mountains, most rice farming is in flooded fields in the high rainfall zones along the western Ghats, in the lower Ganges and Brahmaputra valleys, and in the Himalayas to their north. Rice land in Nepal is about 21 percent irrigated, the rest being rain fed, with spectacular terraced fields on the steep Himalayan slopes. In Bangladesh, the crop is watered by the annual floods of the summer monsoon season, and floating rice of comparatively low yield is often grown. The winter is nearly rainless, but in recent years extensive cultivation of a winter rice crop has been introduced by using high-yielding varieties irrigated with pumped water or planted in areas that remain wet because they are at sea level. Sri Lanka is geographically divided into wet and dry zones. The former is the mountainous two-thirds of the island, which receives heavy rain in the summer monsoon; here rice is generally grown in the lower parts of mountain valleys, in terraced fields watered by direct rain and small rain-fed streams. The dry zone is an area of ancient large-scale reservoir and canal systems, abandoned in the thirteenth century, which have recently been largely restored. Rice fields in this area are irrigated by a combination of large government canals and village-level, rain-fed storage tanks closely akin to those in southern India.

Southeast Asian countries—mainly Burma, Thailand, and Vietnam—are traditional rice exporters. Like Bangladesh, they have large areas of rice irrigated by rainfall and by inundation as the monsoon-fed rivers rise out of their banks. Unlike Bangladesh, their production has historically been relatively high

Brown Rice
Badami Rung

This recipe uses Patna rice, a long-grain white rice, originating in the Bihar region of the Ganges plains. This preparation method is popular in India and Pakistan.

Serves 6

Ingredients
6 tablespoons (90 ml) oil
1 onion, finely chopped
1 pound (450 g) Patna rice or any other long-grain white rice
2 teaspoons (12 g) salt

Preparation
1. In a large skillet, heat the oil over medium heat and fry the onion in the fat until brown, then add the rice and fry for another 10 minutes.

2. In a saucepan, bring 1 quart (1 L) water to a boil. Pour in the rice, fat, fried onion, and enough salt to flavor. Lower the flame and cook very gently until the rice is tender; keep a lid on the pan and test grains of rice for doneness from time to time. Cook on a very low flame; otherwise the rice is apt to burn.

Source: Sri Owen. (1994). *The rice book: The definitive book on rice, with hundreds of exotic recipes from around the world*. New York: St. Martin's Press.

Steamed Plain Rice
Chelo

This is an Iranian recipe, and as the author of the article on Iranian cuisine, M. R. Ghanoon-parvar explains, "rice cooked atop the stove will form a golden crust, the *tahdig*, which can be removed and served in one piece by soaking the bottom of the pot, with the lid closed, in cold water for a few minutes. A good *tahdig* is savored as proof of one's culinary abilities! If you use a nonstick pot, soaking is not necessary." To make the presentation of the rice extra spectacular, a small portion of the rice can be colored with saffron and sprinkled on top before serving.

Serves 6

▶▶

and their costs relatively low. The Philippines has a combination of large river plains now watered by a combination of canals, flooding, and rainfall, and mountain systems like those of Sri Lanka. Indonesia is similar, with ancient, extensive, and extremely well-managed indigenous systems—on Bali, in particular—watered by locally managed channels from rain-fed mountain-top reservoirs.

Ingredients
3 cups (600 g) long- or extra-long-grain rice
4 tablespoons (72 g) salt
¼ cup (60 g) butter, melted, plus more as needed
⅛ teaspoon saffron, dissolved in 2 tablespoons (30 ml) warm water (optional)

Preparation

1. Rinse the rice several times in warm water to remove the starch; drain.

2. Bring at least 2 quarts (2 L) water and 2 tablespoons (36 g) salt to a boil in a large pot; the pot should be large enough to allow the rice to roll around freely as the water boils. Add the rice to the boiling water. Boil 5 to 10 minutes (boiling time differs according to the quality of rice and the amount of soaking time), or until the rice grains are no longer crunchy but still quite firm. Stir occasionally to prevent the grains from sticking together.

3. Drain the rice in a colander.

4. Cover the bottom of the large pot with some of the melted butter. Sprinkle the rice, a large spoonful at a time, into the pot, heaping it at the center so as not to touch the sides of the pot.

5. With the handle of a wooden spoon, perforate the rice in several places all the way to the bottom of the pot and pour in the rest of the melted butter evenly (more melted butter can be added if desired.) Cover the underside of the pot lid with a dish towel (to absorb the moisture that would otherwise accumulate and drip back into the rice, making it soggy) and place the lid tightly on the pot. Cook for approximately 10 minutes over medium heat, then reduce the heat and allow the rice to steam for another 30 minutes or so. The heat can then be turned very low and the rice kept warm until serving time. Rice can also be steamed in a moderate oven for 30 minutes, then turned low until serving time.

6. For decoration, if desired, mix about ⅔ cup (135 g) of the cooked rice with the dissolved saffron so that the rice picks up the color evenly. When the plain rice has been placed on a serving platter, sprinkle the saffron-flavored rice over the top and serve.

Source: M. R. Ghanoonparvar. (2006). *Persian cuisine: Traditional, regional, and modern foods*. Costa Mesa, CA: Mazda Publishers.

In East Asia, rice cultivation is mostly irrigated. In China and Korea, it is more than 91 percent irrigated, while in Japan it is entirely irrigated, although this is mainly in river valleys that have always been naturally wet and subject to flooding. Rice cultivation is commonly combined with fish- or shrimp-raising. Chinese, Korean, and Japanese irrigation systems are recognized as very efficiently managed.

Farm-Level Management

Rice production requires complex social discipline. Throughout Asia, this has consistently involved social systems with strong independent family units operating in the context of close interfamily cooperation at several higher levels. Rice has been essentially a crop of family farmers with small, intensively cultivated holdings that have not lent themselves to mechanization or economies of scale. Most Asian rice farms are three hectares or less, and a very large part of their output is either consumed on the farm or paid out in local wages.

As a rule, family farmers everywhere try to organize their cropping so as to avoid sharp peaks in labor demand that require the heavy use of hired labor. For most crops, this is done by planting several crops each season with different planting, weeding, and harvest times. The ecology of rice militates against this. It precludes other crops, because very few can grow in the conditions rice requires, and a common system of water management requires rice fields to be located side by side over large areas so that water can flow through them. Consequently, a given block of farmers often plants the same rice varieties at substantially the same times. This necessarily means that the labor requirements all tend to peak at about the same time, creating intense local labor shortages. The result is that in rice-growing areas, an extremely large portion of the population is made up of non-landowning agricultural laborers; they are, however, exceptionally well organized, and their wages are usually relatively high. Alternatively, in East Asia, particularly in Japan, where rural labor has become extremely scarce, it is common to replace wage labor with agreements for cooperative labor exchange among landowners, who work in teams on one another's fields.

The high labor demand is mainly for four sets of operations: weeding if the fields are not flooded, transplanting of seedlings if fields are flooded, harvest, and threshing and milling. Transplanting must be done in a short period, because if seedlings are too young they are unlikely to survive, and if they are too mature yields will decline. It is most commonly done by teams of women. Harvesting is most commonly done by hired labor of both sexes, since this is the period of greatest labor scarcity. Payment to the team may be anywhere from a tenth to a sixth of the crop.

Threshing and milling are more difficult with rice, as the husks cling to the individual rice grains more tightly than do other grains. The husks must be removed in a further operation after the grain is separated from the stalk, leaving brown rice. Brown rice is superior in nutrient content to white (milled) rice, but the bran layer that gives it its color contains oils that decompose within a few weeks, spoiling the grain. For long-term storage, unless it is possible to dry the paddy to about 14 percent moisture content, this layer must be removed by milling. In some areas, the rice is also parboiled. Milling was formerly done by pounding the unhusked rice in wooden mortars, usually by the women of a household. Now it is often mechanized. Rice husks are commonly used for fuel and as an abrasive. The bran is a high-quality livestock feed, while the straw is used for fodder, fuel, basketry, and thatch.

Social Implications

In general, the inter-household cooperative arrangements involved in rice production have two major functions: securing resources as needed and managing infrastructure. There are two main patterns.

In areas where rice land makes up only part of total village lands, there is commonly a village reservoir or other water source. The rice lands are those below the reservoir, while higher ground is used for complementary crops. In this case, cooperative arrangements include provisions for maintaining the irrigation infrastructure and distributing the water and also very often for reducing rice plantings in years of low water in such a way as to assure that all those with a right to the water get the use of a proportional section of the land.

In areas where large irrigation systems completely surround whole villages, especially where water flows from one farmer's fields to another's, there must be complex agreements on cropping and water flows below the outlets, as well as on taking turns accessing water from the channels. In East Asia, these arrangements are mainly under farmer control. In South Asia, the larger channels are always controlled by national or provincial officials; farmer responsibility begins at the level of the minor watercourse only, and coordination between the two levels is often poor. In the Philippines, systems were initially built and run as in South Asia. In 1976, however, the National Irrigation Authority nearly went bankrupt. Since then, it has reorganized in such a way as to allow local-level officials to make binding arrangements for construction and management with farmers, which allows the farmers to control what is done and how it is to be paid for, and this system has been a great success.

Hybrid Rice Research in China

Yuan Longping (b. 1930), a Chinese agricultural researcher, started his scientific experiments involving crop cultivation, breeding, and genetics in the 1950s. It wasn't until a decade later, however, with the widespread famine that hit China (1960–1963) following the disastrous policies of the Great Leap Forward (1958–1960), that he began his research on hybrid rice. Observing the results of hybridization in corn, Yuan developed the idea of using hybrids to increase rice yield, but his earliest research efforts met with little success.

In 1970, Yuan and his research team finally discovered a natural male-sterile wild rice plant in Hainan (an island off the coast of southeast China). This led to rapid progress in the development of hybrid rice. Yuan and his team succeeded in breeding unique genetic tools, which consisted of a three-line system (male-sterile line, maintaining line, and restore line) essential for developing high-yielding hybrid rice. Experimental planting was carried out in 1975, and in 1976 the species was made available for widespread use by Chinese farmers. In 1995, Yuan and his team made further advances by developing a two-line system of hybrid rice that promised even higher yields.

The impact on production in China and other parts of the world has been dramatic. For example, in China, rice production increased from three tons per hectare in the late 1960s to nearly seven tons per hectare in 2013. Internationally, Yuan's hybrid rice has been adopted in over twenty other countries, allowing rice yields to increase and keep up with the growing population.

Source: Sullivan, L. R. (2015). Yuan Longping. In Kerry Brown (Ed.), *Berkshire dictionary of Chinese biography* (vol. 4, pp. 517–520). Great Barrington, MA: Berkshire Publishing Group.

Increasing Production

Asian rice production has so far kept pace with increases in population. This is mainly because of the expansion of irrigation and national and international research programs that have introduced new varieties with higher yields (see sidebar on hybrid rice), faster maturation, and greater responsiveness to fertilizer inputs. Expanded irrigation and faster maturation allow farmers to go from one crop per year to two or even three. Until recently, intensification and greater areas planted in rice have been the major sources of increased production. Further gains, however, will have to come more from increased yields.

In the twentieth century, total Asian rice production increased from about 49.38 million metric tons in 1911 to about 540 million metric tons in 1999, and to over 668 million metric tons in 2013. Average yields increased from 1.78 metric tons per hectare in 1930 to over 3.9 tons in 1999, and nearly 4.6 tons in 2013 (FAO 2015). Yet much more is needed: malnutrition is still endemic, poverty is an important constraint on food intake, and population is still increasing.

Hope lies in the fact that rice yields, along with yields of other grains, can rise well above present levels. This has often been demonstrated experimentally, but more important, it is also evident in the great variations in productivity within and between countries, ranging from 3.0 tons/hectare in Cambodia through 3.6 in India to 6.7 in China and the Republic of Korea (FAO 2015). While some of these differences may reflect natural conditions, the more likely explanation lies in farmers' differing access to resources, and this can readily be improved.

Murray J. LEAF

University of Texas at Dallas

Further Reading

Barker, R.; Herdt, R. W.; & Rose, B. (1985). *The rice economy of Asia*. Washington, DC: Resources for the Future.

Food and Agricultural Organization of the United Nations (FAO). (2015). FAOStat. Retrieved April 22, 2015, from http://faostat3.fao.org/browse/Q/QC/E

Lansing, J. S. (1991). *Priests and programmers: Technologies of power in the engineered landscape of Bali.* Princeton, NJ: Princeton University Press.

Leaf, M. J. (1998). *Pragmatism and development: The Prospect for pluralist transformation in the third world*. New York: Bergin and Garvey.

Randhawa, M. S. (1980–1986). *A history of agriculture in India* (4 vols.). New Delhi: Indian Council of Agricultural Research.

Yuan, L. (1996). Hybrid rice in China. In Directorate of Rice Research (Eds.), *Hybrid rice technology* (51–54 pp.). Hyderabad: India.

Tofu

First prepared in China, tofu has become one of the mainstays of Asian cooking, especially for countries where Buddhism has been pervasive. Made from soybeans that are boiled and compressed, tofu is a nutritious and easily available food source and is often added to spicy sauces, where it soaks up flavors.

One of the great breakthroughs in human nutrition was the discovery of how to process difficult-to-digest soybeans into nutritious tofu, or *doufu* 豆腐 in Chinese. Tofu is made by soaking soybeans overnight, grinding them finely with water, and boiling them into a slurry, filtered to produce soy milk. This can then be precipitated using various settlers, commonly magnesium salts, Japanese *okara*, and pressed into slabs. It is uncertain when tofu was first made, but the technology was well known in China by early medieval times and possibly as early as the Han dynasty (206 BCE–220 CE). Imitation of cheese-making as practiced in the Altaic region has been cited as one possible source of the idea. The technology of tofu-making is both similar to and different from Altaic cheese-making, which strives to produce a durable, usually dried product (e.g., Kazakh *qurt*), whereas tofu is usually used fresh—although it can be dried—and, of course, Altaic cheese is never prepared from anything other than milk. The modern Mongols and Turks thus have not acquired a taste for tofu, except perhaps in Inner Mongolia with its heavily Sinified foodways. An alternative interpretation to the cheese-imitation theory is that tofu originated in Daoist macrobiotic experiments.

Tofu in Asia

The early history of tofu in China is obscure, and tofu is rarely mentioned in cookbooks and agricultural manuals which, in any case, appeared late in China. What is known is that tofu seems to have begun its rise to near universality as a meat substitute as monk's food. In Vietnam, where Buddhism is still more of

124

Japanese Tofu Scones

Many people still think of tofu (bean curd) as a bland ingredient used primarily by vegetarians as a meat replacement. These Japanese tofu "scones" might not be the most typical tofu dish, but it does show the extremely versatile nature of this soy product.

In the original Japanese cookbook, these scones are described as a sweet snack, a light bread that would be served with preserves. It is literally titled *tofu bread*, but the picture looks more like a fluffy biscuit or a scone. This recipe also works great as a platform for other flavors, either a sweetener such as honey, or a savory one such as grated Parmesan. Add these as desired to the exceedingly simple basic recipe.

Ingredients
½ cup (100 g) extra-firm tofu, crumbled
½ to ⅔ cup (55 to 85 g) all-purpose flour
1 teaspoon baking powder
Pinch of salt
Few drops of sesame oil (optional)
Milk, egg wash, or vegetable oil (optional)
Sesame seeds (optional)

Preparation
1. Preheat the oven to 350°F (175°C). Line a baking sheet with parchment paper.

2. In a large bowl, mix together the tofu, flour, baking powder, salt, and sesame oil by hand or using a hand mixer. Continue to knead the dough until it starts to come together, 5 to 10 minutes. If at first the dough appears to be crumbling and falling apart, be patient; keep kneading until the dough becomes firmer and holds together.

3. Cut out the scones, either free-form or using a round cookie or biscuit cutter. Brush the top of the scones with some milk, egg wash, or vegetable oil. Sprinkle with sesame seeds.

4. Bake the scones for 15 to 20 minutes, or until a toothpick inserted in the middle comes out clean and the scones are a golden-brown color on the top. These are best served warm, with either sweet (honey, butter and marmalade, compote) or savory (cream cheese, chili jam, or even pesto) condiments.

Source: Recipe adapted by Thomas DuBois (https://thomasdaviddubois.wordpress.com/2017/10/10/recipe-review-tofu-scones/) from the Japanese cookbook *Yasai no gohan*, with further adjustments by Marjolijn Kaiser.

a force than in China, Buddhist festivals are marked with huge monk-food feasts where tofu and tofu skin, *doufupi*, are modeled and flavored into meat substitutes of every kind, from fish to fowl. The tradition continues not only in Asia but in the Western world, where vegans and others with vegetarian interests use tofu and tofu products in much the same way.

Whether it was first originally a monk's food or not, probably no later than the Song dynasty (960–1279), tofu became a standard ingredient for Chinese high cuisine as well (about the same time, it also began to gain popularity in other Buddhist countries like Japan and Vietnam). A typical dish, although the form eaten today probably dates long after the Song, is *mapo doufu*, "hemp woman bean curd," although the meaning of the name is uncertain and the *po* is perhaps a transcription of some local word. Although designated as a Sichuan dish, the recipe is actually from Hunan. It is cooked in a wok and starts with peanut oil in which sliced pork is cooked with shallots, chilies, garlic, and ginger—the latter three a typical spicing combination. Added to that is the sliced tofu along with black mushrooms and green onions, thinly sliced, and soy sauce to add taste, lightly. When the mixture is cooked and ready to eat, a few tablespoons of refined sesame oil is added, and on top of that ground Chinese flower pepper—the signature spice of the dish. Firm tofu is used, and cooks are careful not to use too much oil. In Korea, a characteristic dish is *toenjang tubu tchigae*. In its base form, it is a soup made with Korean hot bean paste, *toenjang*; a small amount of pork is an option and perhaps some additional garlic or ginger (many other additions are possible to make a stew, even anchovies) and tofu. It is spicy and nutritious.

In Vietnam, other than the pervasive monk's food, tofu is used much as in China, including for stir fries—though less so in soups, in which pressed blood is often used in much the same role, a favorite being beef soup in the Hue style, *bún bò Huế*. In Japan, tofu is less likely to be spicy as it is often served in China, but is a typical part of Japanese miso soup and is even served on its own with a sprinkle of salt and chopped chives.

In recent times, and since the Song, tofu has become a mainstay of Chinese cooking and is a cheap and easily accessible source of protein. Nonetheless, in spite of its importance, tofu remains underrepresented in the classic cookbooks, but this may be due to its plebeian origins. Other tofu products include, as noted above and which is very important in monk's food, the "skin," *doufupi*, skimmed off and dried during the cooking process; and *choudoufu*, "stinking bean curd," a fermented product that is an acquired taste much loved in Taiwan. From a commercial standpoint, the poor man's food tofu has the added advantage, besides its nutritional value, of being easily produced and generally available—anywhere the soybean grows. This means no politics when it comes to soybeans as a food product, unlike the case with rice, where efforts are made to control the trade for commercial advantage and dominance.

Paul D. BUELL

University of North Georgia

Further Reading

Anderson, E. N. (1988). *The food of China*. New Haven, CT: Yale University Press.

Huang, H. T. (2000). *Biology and biological technology*. Science and Civilization in China series. Cambridge, UK: Cambridge University Press.

Huang, H. T. (2000). *Fermentations and food science*. Science and Civilization in China series. Cambridge, UK: Cambridge University Press.

Shurtleff, W. & Aoyagi, A. (1975). *The book of tofu*. Berkeley, CA: Ten Speed Press.

Tea: East Asia

Tea and tea drinking have become synonymous with Asian culture, with China being the most dominant in its production and cultivation. The habit of drinking tea, first as a medicinal draught and then as a beverage, spread from China to Japan and Korea and eventually west to the Middle East, Europe, and the Americas.

Tea is the leaf, bud, and twig of *Camellia sinensis* and was probably first domesticated in Southeast Asia, although a number of possible sites have been named, including some in South China. There are several varieties; some, such as Assam tea from India, are quite distinctive. Tea is cultivated at moderate altitudes in tropical and semi-tropical areas, usually in marginal soils not suited to growing highly productive food crops such as rice. There are two main kinds of tea on the market today: black tea ("red tea" in Chinese), and green tea, not as highly processed as black tea, which is "fermented," that is, oxidized. The popular oolong tea is a variety of black tea, relatively less fermented, and traded widely. There are many other variants including "white tea," a term which covers a number of varieties of minimally processed teas and parts of the tea plant.

A third type of tea found in Central Asia, including Tibet, is brick tea. This is an oxidized tea compressed into brick form. For drinking, it is boiled for a long time in whole, fresh milk or cream. This product is "milk tea," the Mongolian *suutay tsai*, "tea with milk," the normal beverage offered to guests in Central Asia. Brick tea is regularly fortified with parched barley and butter to make *tsampa*, a food as well as a drink.

Tea is normally prepared in one of two ways: through infusion (dipping tea leaves into hot water) or by dissolving the leaves, after they have been ground into a powder, in hot water. Central Asian tea preparation is a variant of the former. In Vietnam and Korea, where tea seems to have arrived late, only in the seventh century, tea is prepared much as in China: through infusion. The Japanese prefer making most of their tea from powder, although this is not always done with green tea. Korea has a significant tea substitute in its roasted barely tea, *bon cha*. Herb teas are also particularly popular in Korea, but apparently little green tea was consumed in traditional times. The role of tea in ancestral rites is particularly important in Korea and has been for centuries.

Tea in China

Initially, tea was a rare medicinal in China, but by Song times (960–1279) it had become a common beverage, a huge commercial property, and the basis of a complete cultural experience. By Southern Song times (1125–1279) it was grown in the hilly areas of Fujian and neighboring Jiangxi, but its cultivation was later expanded to other suitable areas. Its cultivation was later established in Yunnan, for example, when Yunnan definitely became a part of China during Yuan and Ming times. Fine tea is still grown there, including some of the most famous varieties such as *pu'er*, which comes in "camel pellets," small prepared doses. From China, tea drinking spread to the West, at first as a medicinal drink and then, with the appearance of the Mongols, a beverage. There are today many variants, not just Central Asian milk tea, but specially cultivated teas in the Middle East and Turkey, for example.

TEA DRINKING

Tea drinking as such arose in China around the beginning of our era but was at first a localized practice and confined to the south, then barely Chinese. Only gradually did tea, at first brewed from green leaves, become more a recreational beverage than a pure medicinal. By the Tang dynasty (618–906) the practice had become general, south and north—but tea as a growth industry fueling the economy came later. During the Song dynasty, tea drinking became the rage, as it has continued to be down to the present. Song tea was a product greatly in demand, not only in China but among Tibetans and other neighbors of China—and later, from the eleventh and twelfth centuries on, even in the far West. It is mentioned in the medical work of the great Ibn Sīnā (980–1137) of Persia, for example. By Southern Song times, tea had become an economic powerhouse and a primary basis for the prosperity of the dynasty. In the West, the real rise of tea as an economic force came with the British acquisition of India and its tea resources, although Chinese tea was traded too. This is shown by the English word tea, from the local Fujian pronunciation *te*—as opposed to the north Chinese and Cantonese *cha*, the form that is the basis for Mongolian *tsai* and the ubiquitous Central Asian and Iranian *shay* or *chai* (to say nothing of the British slang *cha*).

Although the first teas were leaf, the preferred form of tea during Tang times was brick tea, now more or less obsolete except in Central Asia and along China's Central Asian borders zones. This used large square bricks of pressed tea leaves boiled for long periods of time to produce a strong and thick beverage consumed with milk and cream. Later, particularly under the Song, powdered teas became common; this was the form of tea later taken over by Japan as the basis for its tea ceremony. By late Song times, carefully selected leaf teas had also become common, and these were associated with a substantial connoisseurship. More recently, oxidized leaf and pressed teas, known incorrectly as fermented teas (though some teas actually have been fermented) have been popular and were long the preferred form of tea for the European and American export market. But these were already Chinese teas before foreigners began buying them (although the story is told by the Chinese that stupid foreigners started buying the "fermented" teas because they were too stupid to know when the teas in question were spoiled. The story that a shipload of tea rotted and that Europeans, not knowing any better, liked the flavor of the rotten tea, although entertaining, is—alas—folklore. Some of the oxidized teas are even highly regarded in China to this day, the Yunnan teas for example).

Culture of Tea

There never was anything quite comparable to the Japanese tea ceremony in China (or for that matter Vietnam and Korea), but there was a distinct culture of tea beginning during the period of disunity and continuing to be popular many centuries thereafter. Playing a key role in the development of this tea culture were Buddhist monasteries and monks. Like the Sufis who helped introduce their favorite beverage of coffee to the Islamic world, Buddhist monks seem to have enjoyed tea as a stimulant during dull monastic work or even meditation. Probably because of this practice, tea drinking became a formal part of monastic rituals, which helped to stress the elegance, simplicity, and introspection involved. Since monasteries were never isolated from the secular world in medieval and early modern China, laymen soon became involved both in monastic tea culture and their own varieties of it. These were developed outside monasteries but incorporated much of the ritualized content of monastic tea consumption. Tea drinking thus became an important link between the literati and the monastic culture of Zen in particular, and it was an earmark of Song dynasty culture.

Outside both literati culture and the monastery, tea was also consumed during Song times at the tea house. Restaurants as they exist today—and, for that matter, tea houses—first appeared in China. Places where one could go, eat a few snacks, drink tea, and enjoy the company of others (especially female company) were noticed, among others, by Marco Polo. Tea houses were more specialized than restaurants, and from the beginning, the society of the tea house was associated with prostitution, but this did not make them any less popular. Tea houses were already present in the Tang capital of Chang'an in large numbers in the eighth century. During the Five Dynasties and Song periods, tea houses were not only associated with female entertainment but also with a particular form of poetry, the *ci*. These verses were set to popular melodies and usually sung by the women of tea houses and the formal houses of prostitution. During this period, the most famous literati wrote *ci*, although they did not originate the form, and through their verses we know a great deal about the popular houses of the Southern Song capital of Hangzhou, for example.

LITERATURE OF TEA

Going along with a distinct culture of tea was a specialized literature of tea. The most famous work in this genre is the *Chajing* (*Tea Classic*) of Lu Yu, from the late eighth century. His ten-volume work is a compendium of tea lore, including its Taoist connection as a magic herb, the medical qualities of tea itself, its food value, and even descriptions of tea bowls. Other important works on tea include the *Chalu* (*Record of Tea*) of Cai Xiang (1012–1067) and the *Daguan Chalun* (*Discussion of Tea of the Daguan Period*) by the Song emperor Huizong (r. 1101–1125) himself, who was known for his painting, calligraphy, and refined tastes.

PORCELAIN

During Song times, a key dimension of tea culture was porcelain tea bowls, created in special shapes, textures, and colors just for tea drinking. Porcelain is different from other potteries in its raw materials and its very high firing temperatures. Although not invented by the Song, porcelain reached its first high point under that dynasty. The most famous of Song porcelains were celadons. These were created in a blue-green color by applying a thick glaze to a relatively delicate base. Celadon was the preferred porcelain of the court, but the Song period is also known for its black ware, including Jian tea bowls. With these bowls, a black glaze was intended to contrast with the green color of the tea consumed in them. The body of the bowl, relatively thick, helped maintain the temperature of the beverage. Although considered a popular ware, such bowls were still used at court, by the literati, and at monasteries. Fine examples continue to be highly prized today, and Song porcelain was imitated throughout East Asia and beyond. From Mongol times, it was also a trade good, at first overland and then large-scale by sea. No later than the early fourteenth century, Chinese blue and white porcelain, the blue celebrating the sacred color of the Mongols, had reached at least as far as Bulgaria. How much its spread contributed to changing culinary habits, a soupy Mongol-era cuisine, and the spread of tea drinking itself is unclear.

Tea in Japan

Tea was transmitted to Japan in the early ninth century. The emperor and his courtiers in the capital city of Heian-kyō (Kyoto), enamored of China's higher civilization, drank and appreciated tea as an elegant beverage. At Buddhist temples, priests and monks consumed it primarily for their health. Tea drinking largely died out, however, in the late ninth and tenth centuries as the Japanese ended what had been approximately three centuries of cultural borrowing from China. The beverage was reintroduced to Japan in the late twelfth century by the Zen Buddhist priest Eisai (1141–1215), who praised tea as a medicine beneficial to the heart. Eisai also strongly recommended tea as an aid in the Buddhist practice of seated meditation. By the fourteenth century, tea had spread throughout Japan and had become a national drink.

TEA CEREMONY

The Japanese tea ceremony (*chanoyu*) is a ritualized form of preparing and serving tea, usually in a carefully designed and controlled setting known as the tea room (*chashitsu*). The tea ceremony uses green tea in powdered form. After placing powdered tea into a bowl several times larger than the Western tea cup, the host ladles in water and stirs the tea and water into a frothy mixture with a split-bamboo whisk.

The tea ceremony evolved during the fifteenth and sixteenth centuries and reached its high point in the time of Sen no Rikyū (1522–1591), who is universally recognized as the greatest of the tea masters. In Rikyū's day, the leading tea masters stood at the apex of Japanese cultural life. They were respected not only as skilled performers of the ceremony itself but also as men of taste in the various arts associated with the ceremony, including ceramics and lacquerware, room construction and decoration (the masters designed and decorated their own tea rooms), painting, calligraphy, and flower arrangement—all Zen arts. Whereas the tea ceremony was performed almost exclusively by men in premodern times, from the late nineteenth century, it became predominately a female pursuit. The tea ceremony is one of Japan's most enduring arts, and to learn how to handle oneself correctly at a tea ceremony is to acquire the essential features of traditional Japanese etiquette and manners. This is particularly so for young women, the principal students of the tea ceremony in modern times. Through study of the tea ceremony, young women learn how to wear kimonos correctly, how to walk and sit in a kimono, how to serve tea and food properly to guests, and how to conduct themselves with elegance and style.

Tea in Mongolia

Although brick tea was already exported to Tibet under the Tang, tea drinking only began much later as a general Central Asian practice. The earliest reference to traditional Mongolian tea, long-boiled (later brick) tea with thick milk or cream, for example, only dates to the fourteenth century, where an apparent recipe is found in the imperial dietary for Mongol China, the *Yinshan Zhengyao* (*Proper and Essential Things for the Emperor's Food and Drink*), along with many other tea recipes showing the growing popularity of all kinds of teas among the Mongols and other foreigners at court at the time. In addition to its early recipe for Mongolian tea, in this case a powdered tea boiled with liquid butter under a Turkic name—suggesting that the Mongols may have borrowed it from local Turks—that same source mentions many other kinds of tea as being drunk at court, including Jade Mortar Tea, made from tea and roasted rice; Golden Characters Tea, a powdered tea from the south; Mr. Fan Tianshuai's tea, a tribute bud tea from south China; and Purple Shoots Sparrow Tongue Tea, made from new shoots.

With these beginnings, tea caught on in Mongolia, as witnessed by the position of tea in the Ming dynasty's (1368–1644) trade with the north. As had once been done with the Tibetans, Song China's source of horses, the Ming traded masses of tea to the Mongols in exchange for ponies. In Mongolia itself, tea quickly became a way of life. Not offering a visitor tea became unthinkable, and Mongols, like Tibetans, also added barley and other ingredients to their tea along with butter, to provide a hot staple that is still consumed today. Mongolian tea, in fact, with or without millet and butter, is a wonderful beverage and just what is called for on a cold day.

Tea Beyond East Asia

Tea consumption spread west to Iran (then known as Persia), then the Turkish world, and finally Europe. From as early as the tenth century, tea was thought to be medicinal in Iran; it has now become the drink of choice with many local variants, with a preference for black tea. In Turkey, tea drinking took hold, but after the sixteenth century, coffee became the beverage of choice, although it never entirely eliminated tea drinking. Since Chinese tea bowls were preferred in many areas of the West, the tea cultures of Iran and Turkey were not that different from that of China.

Europe too took up tea drinking, influenced by the Islamic world, as Europeans later did with coffee. The Western world's coffee was from Cairo, but Europe still obtained most of its tea from China, as did the North American colonies. Although Britain tried to push the teas of India, where tea was domesticated and developed independently of China, Chinese teas continued to be imported both to Britain and elsewhere in Europe, leading to a vast trading crisis as European silver went east to pay for Chinese tea, the first true mass commodity of the European trading system, if we exclude slaves. The attempt by Britain to substitute Indian opium for silver to cut its costs ultimately led to a series of wars with China, but the tea trade continued right down to the present, when Chinese teas are making a come-back on the world market. This is even the case in spite of the fact that coffee has been of growing importance in Europe and America since the eighteenth century, when Bach wrote his "Coffee Cantata" to celebrate its use. Even Vietnam has taken up drinking and producing coffee of very high quality. But coffee, in spite of the high quality Turkish coffee produced by the Turks (and Arabs) and the derivative expresso, simply lacks the delicacy of tea (and coffee drinking lacks the simplicity and elegance of tea drinking)—thus its continued importance throughout the world.

Paul D. BUELL (China, Mongolia, and beyond East Asia)

University of North Georgia

Paul VARLEY (Japan)

Columbia University

Further Reading

Buell, Paul D.; Anderson, E. N.; & Perry, C. (2010). *A soup for the Qan: Chinese dietary medicine of the Mongol era as seen in Hu Szu-hui's Yinshan zhengyao* (2nd ed.). Leiden and Boston: E. J. Brill.

Anderson, E. N.; Perry, C.; & de Pablo, M. (Eds.). (Forthcoming 2017). *Crossroads of cuisine: The Eurasian heartland, the Silk Roads and food.* London: Prospect Books.

Ludwig, T. (1981). Before Rikyu. Religious and aesthetic influences in the early history of the tea ceremony. *Monumenta Nipponica, 36*(4), 367–390.

Suzuki, D. T. (1959). *Zen and Japanese culture.* Princeton: Princeton University Press (Bollingen Series LXIV).

Anderson, J. L. (1991). *An introduction to Japanese tea ritual.* Albany, NY: State University of New York Press.

Hirota, D. (Ed.). (1995). *Wind in the pines.* Fremont, CA: Asian Humanities Press.

Sadler, A. L. (1962). *Cha-no-yu, the Japanese tea ceremony.* Tokyo: Tuttle.

Sen S. (1998). *The Japanese way of tea.* Honolulu, HI: University of Hawaii Press.

Varley, P. & Isao Kumakura (Eds.). (1989). *Tea in Japan: Essays on the history of chanoyu.* Honolulu, HI: University of Hawaii Press.

Tea: South Asia

South Asia is one of the most important producers, exporters, and consumers of tea. Since the nineteenth century and the rise of tea plantations in India and Sri Lanka, tea has become one of the defining characteristics of South Asia, with each country of the subcontinent putting its own spin on how tea is prepared and enjoyed.

Although tea (*Camellia sinensis*) is native to China, much of tea production shifted to South Asia in the first half of the nineteenth century. In 1998, South Asia was the most important producer and exporter of tea (accounting for 30.3 percent and 38.8 percent, respectively). A massive workforce, about 1.5 million people, is engaged in tea production in South Asia, and tea is responsible for a considerable, though declining, share of export earnings for the producing countries. Tea is produced in about twenty-five countries, the most important (outside South Asia) being China, Kenya, Turkey, and Indonesia. The main consumers are (in descending order of consumption) Russia, the United Kingdom, the United States, and Egypt. Tea is produced in three main varieties: as orthodox tea (the main producer is Sri Lanka), as CTC-tea (where the leaf is cut, torn, and curled before firing/heating; the main producers are India and Kenya), and as green tea (manufactured without firing; the main producer is China).

Tea Culture

In South Asia, a large and growing proportion of tea is consumed internally (in India, more than two-thirds of production) as a popular and extremely cheap drink (often prepared on the road in "tea stalls" by *chai wallahs*) and sold most often in packets, very rarely in bags or as iced tea. In Indian homes, tea will always be offered to guests, and is frequently prepared with milk, sugar, and spices such as cardamom, black pepper, and cinnamon, known as masala chai. Sri Lankans also drink tea at home, though it is most likely to be black tea

136

with sugar and warm milk. In Pakistan, black or green tea is made into a strong brew and is enjoyed in the morning, during afternoon tea breaks, and in the evening with sweet snacks. Kashmiris indulge in a rich brew known as noon chai, very milky and infused with pistachios and cardamom, during the winter months and for special occasions. As in other regions of South Asia, tea brings Pakistanis together for everything from business meetings, to marriage proposals, to many other social occasions.

India

In India, tea production began in 1838 and slowly spread from Assam (still the most important tea-growing area) to other parts of north India and later to south India (the Nilgiri Hills). First planted by individual farmers, tea quickly became a company business owned by British firms, which withdrew from the subcontinent (especially in the 1950s and 1960s) only because of declining tea prices, growing labor unrest, strict (government-imposed) social obligations (to provide employees with free housing, schooling, health care, and so on), and narrow ceilings on foreign ownership.

Most Indian tea is produced on big plantations; small landholders play a role only in south India. Although India is responsible for nearly 30 percent of world tea production, it accounts for only 16 percent of world exports, as an increasing proportion is consumed locally. The government has often intervened in tea exportation by setting export quotas to protect local consumers (tea is treated as an essential commodity), by restricting plantations' land acquisition and use through land reform acts, and by imposing heavy taxes on tea companies. The Indian tea industry is in a healthy condition (apart from a few "sick gardens" taken over by the government), and productivity per hectare is very high. Nonetheless, in 2001, south Indian wholesale prices of five rupees per kilogram made tea production unprofitable for small producers.

Sri Lanka and Bangladesh

In Sri Lanka, tea production began in 1867. Individual planters were soon replaced by British companies, which managed their estates by means of local agency houses. Fieldwork and picking were carried out by an immigrant workforce that arrived in large numbers from south India until the Indian colonial government called a halt to the emigrations in the 1930s. The state has supported the expansion of the plantation system by taking over land to which nobody could provide a legal title, providing infrastructure, and ensuring generous tax treatment.

Independence in 1948 led to almost immediate revolt against the plantation system, escalating export taxes, government interference, and finally (in 1972 and 1975) nationalization of the tea estates, which were brought under two state corporations. Their unsatisfactory performance slowly paved the way for privatization of management in 1992 and for full privatization after 1996. Sri Lanka has lost export market shares and its reputation for tea quality until recently; since privatization, performance is improving.

Bangladesh is responsible for only 1.9 percent of world tea production and consumes 60 percent of its own production.

The Future

Tea was once the pillar of India's and Sri Lanka's export economy and as such an easy target of anticolonial agitation. Since independence, tea has lost much of its former economic importance in these countries. The falling relevance of tea exports (but not consumption) for South Asia could not have been avoided, because world consumption is increasing very slowly, causing tea prices (in real terms) to stagnate or decline.

Joachim BETZ

German Institute for Global and Area Studies (GIGA)

Further Reading

Betz, J. (1993). *Agrarische Rohstoffe und Entwicklung: Teewirtschaft und Teeproduktion in Sri Lanka, Indien, und Kenia* (Agricultural raw materials and development: Tea business and tea production in Sri Lanka, India, and Kenya). Hamburg, Germany: German Overseas Institute.

De Silva, S. B. D. (1982). *The political economy of underdevelopment*. London: Routledge and Keagan.

Forrest, D. (1985). *The world tea trade*. Cambridge, UK: Woodhead-Faulkner.

Rote, R. (1986). *A taste of bitterness: The political economy of tea plantations in Sri Lanka*. Amsterdam: Free University Press.

Spice Trade

The preservative, medicinal, and seasoning qualities of tropical spices, like cinnamon, ginger, and pepper, sparked intense trafficking in spices across oceans and continents even before the beginning of the Christian Era. During the European Age of Discovery, the islands of Southeast Asia became the geographical center of this trade.

Most spices are native to the tropical and subtropical regions of South and Southeast Asia. Spices such as salt, saffron, pepper, ginger, cardamom, nutmeg, clove, and cinnamon have, since time immemorial, been highly valued as medicines, ointments, aphrodisiacs, stimulants, antiseptics, and preservatives. Their use as seasonings for various dishes or ingredients for incenses and oils predates recorded history. The ancient recognition of the therapeutic value of salt, for instance, resonates through the etymology of the Latin words *salus* ("bliss") and *salubritas* ("health"), which are derived from the Latin word *sal* ("salt"). In the European Middle Ages, pepper and salt were widely used as preservatives for meat. The healing and stimulating capacities of spices like ginger, nutmeg, and cardamom contributed to the fact that in various ancient cultures, such as those of early China and India, cooking was regarded as a sacred act.

During the European Age of Discovery, the Moluccas, now part of Indonesia, became known as the spice islands par excellence because they were the home of the "holy trinity" of nutmeg, clove, and pepper. Nutmeg and clove were, in fact, native to the Moluccas and had not been transplanted to other tropical regions before the arrival of the Europeans in Southeast Asia. Pepper, on the other hand, is said to be indigenous to the Malabar Coast of India, but it had long been cultivated throughout Southeast Asia. Sumatra, for instance, became a favorite destination of European East India merchants for its wealth of pepper. Ginger is probably native to Southeast Asia, but it was already widely known in ancient India and China. Cinnamon, also already widely used in Asian antiquity, originates from Sri Lanka. Cardamom is native to the rain forests of

South India. South India and Sri Lanka were the exclusive areas of its cultivation when Europeans arrived in the Indian Ocean. Saffron, for which India (especially Kashmir) and Northern China have been famous, probably originated in the Mediterranean, the Near East, and Iran. The demand for spices such as pepper, cinnamon, cardamom, ginger, turmeric, saffron, nutmeg, and clove, which were domesticated in South and Southeast Asia, was an important factor in the evolution of long-distance trade.

Spices in Local Cuisines and Medicine

Aside from being lucrative trade goods, these spices have played an important part in the local cuisines and folk medicinal systems of Asian societies. Neolithic stone implements, such as the mortars and rubbing stones exhibited in the Indonesian National Museum in Jakarta, suggest a widespread use of herbs and spices, grinded for daily health and beauty care as well as aphrodisiacal purposes, already in prehistoric times. Reliefs on Borobudur, the famous Central Javanese Buddhist monument from the ninth century CE, depict women pounding leaves from a mythological tree together with other ingredients to produce cosmetics and medicine. Classical Javanese literature, too, refers to the medicinal benefits of a whole range of spices. The eighteenth century Javanese text *Serat Centhini*, for instance, recommends chewing ylang-ylang (*canagium odoratum*) flowers, mixed with salt, as a treatment for toothache. Natural medicine, called *jamu* in present-day Java, is still produced by women in rural areas. Turmeric and ginger are popular ingredients in these medicinal concoctions. Ginger is believed to stimulate the appetite, to aid digestion, and to help alleviate rheumatic pain. Turmeric, for its part, has for ages been used for coloring dishes, as yellow is traditionally considered to be a sacred color, symbolizing the sun, light, and energy. Both spices furthermore have enjoyed ample use as food seasonings and preservatives.

Spices have held a similar range of functions in the Chinese five-element cuisine, which distinguishes between five tastes or flavors: sour, bitter, sweet, pungent, and salty. Each of these flavors is incidentally ascribed to a whole range of different spices, plants, and herbs. Pepper, chili, garlic, ginger, coriander, star anise, mandarin peel, clove, fennel seeds, mustard greens, and cassia are all associated with the pungent taste, for instance, which in practice is thus much more nuanced than the simple five-flavor scheme at first suggests.

Spice Trade

Given their longstanding diversified use and value, it should not come as a surprise that the spice trade reaches back far into prehistoric times. Around 2000

BCE, different spice routes had already reached the Middle East. Many references to the early Arabian trade in spices are to be found in the Bible (for example, Joseph was sold to a group of Ishmaelite spice merchants on their way to Egypt). In the fourth century BCE, the Greek historian Herodotus wrote that wild animals and steep cliffs render the spice gardens, lying somewhere in the distant East, inaccessible. His account was inspired by the stories of Arab traders, who tried to withhold the true origins of their highly prized goods.

One of the trade routes for spices was actually the Silk Road, connecting ancient China and India with Parthia (i.e., present-day Iran), Arabia, and the Levant. After the Emperor Han Wudi (156–87 BCE) had extended the Great Wall to the Yumen Pass, near Dunhuang, and had put in place a system of garrisons, the international merchants travelling the Silk Road enjoyed much greater safety. From Yungang in today's Shanxi Province to Bamiyan in central Afghanistan, Buddhist monasteries nestled along the entire Central Asian part of the Silk Road, providing shelter for most travelers.

Powerful Arab merchants controlled the commerce with the Greeks, Parthians, and Romans, dominating not only the land but also the profitable sea routes, along which spices and fragrances from India, Africa, and Arabia were traded to the Mediterranean. In the first century CE, the Romans succeeded in breaking the Arabian monopoly on the trade with India for several centuries. Yet, after the fall of Rome in the sixth century, the Arab monopoly over the spice trade was quickly restored. The land as well as sea routes to the East soon also functioned as conduits for the new Arab religion, Islam, propagated in the seventh century by Muhammad (c. 570–632), who had married a widow of a wealthy Arabian spice merchant.

The threshold to the European market, on the other hand, was guarded by Christian Byzantium. In 1204, however, it was sacked by Venice, its economic rival, which then became the Western trade center for spices until the sixteenth century.

In 1260, the Venetian merchants Nicolo and Mafeo Polo travelled along the Silk Road to the court of Kublai Khan, whence they returned to Venice in 1269. In 1271, they embarked on a second journey to the Yuan emperor's court, together with their son and nephew, the then only fifteen-year-old Marco. When they finally reached the Yuan court, they were to remain in Kublai Khan's entourage for twenty years before they were allowed to return home. In his book, *Il Milione*, Marco Polo frequently mentioned places rich in spices, like the island of Zipangu in the South China Sea abounding in pepper, lignum-aloes, trees with fragrant blossoms, and so forth. Very often he referred to spices in conjunction with local wines and liquors as well as perfumes. In Cathay, for instance, people would drink rice wine mixed with spices and drugs. Similarly, in Tibet, people would drink a very tasty wine made from a mixture of wheat, rice, and spices.

When in 1368 the Yuan dynasty was overthrown by a massive rebellion, which eventually led to the establishment of the Ming dynasty, the Mongols retreated into the steppe, and the Silk Road began to decline. The caravan towns and the religious facilities supporting them were gradually abandoned and finally covered by desert sands.

Manju's Curry Powder
Manju Ka Masala

Creating your own curry spice blend is perhaps the best way to get a sense of South Asian flavors. This recipe comes from a cookbook designed for modern cooks who want quick and simple dishes with authentic flavors.

Ingredients
6 dried red chilies
¼ teaspoon black peppercorns
5 cloves
2 or 3 green cardamom pods
¼ teaspoon cumin seeds
¼ teaspoon coriander seeds
2 small pieces cassia bark or cinnamon
¼ teaspoon ground turmeric

Preparation
1. Heat a heavy skillet over low heat, then add all of the spices except the turmeric and cook for a couple of minutes to bring out the aroma and flavors, shaking the pan occasionally and being careful not to let the ingredients burn.

2. Remove the pan from the heat and set it aside to cool, then place the spices in a clean coffee or spice grinder with the turmeric and whiz to a fine powder; you may have to do this in batches depending on the size of the grinder. The ground ingredients will have a pungent smell, so be careful when you open the coffee grinder. You will need ½ to 1 teaspoon of this blend to season a dish for four people. Store in an airtight container for up to 6 months.

Note
If you don't have dried red chilies, replace them with 1 teaspoon chili powder, which you can add along with the turmeric to the ground spices.

Source: Manju Malhi. (2002). *Brit spice*. London: Michael Joseph Publishing.

By 1500, European discoverers, seeking to evade the heavy taxes imposed by the Ottomans in the Levant and the Mamelukes in Egypt, had found the sea passage to the spice regions of India, Ceylon (Sri Lanka), Sumatra, and the Moluccas. In the following centuries, several European East India companies competed with each other in monopolizing larger or smaller segments of the spice trade in the Indian Ocean and the South China Sea. From 1600 onward, the most successful merchant associations were the British East India Company and its Dutch equivalent, the Vereenigde Oost-Indische Compagnie, also known as the Dutch East India Company. By the late eighteenth century, however, their spice monopolies were broken due to the successful transplantation of South and Southeast Asian spice plants to other parts of the world.

As a result, exotic spices ceased to be regarded as luxury goods, priceless, and beyond the reach of the common people in Europe. During the middle ages, oriental spices had possessed not only a culinary but also a ceremonial value. The heavily seasoned dishes served at the royal feasts of medieval courts had not only been intended to please the palate of the guests but to underscore the status of their regal host. When in 1194 the King of Scotland paid a visit to Richard I of England, he received from the latter a daily ration of two pounds of pepper and four pounds of cinnamon, which was just as much a sign of favor as an ostentatious display of power. It was in fact a voracious need for spices on the part of the European aristocracy that drove the European Age of Discovery. Interestingly, during the seventeenth century, Europe's aristocracy lost interest in strongly flavored dishes. This change of taste mirrored the sinking status of spices occasioned by the colonial spice trade. At the same time, new colonial goods, such as tea, coffee, chocolate, and sugar, were replacing the oriental spices as markers of high status in European societies.

Martin RAMSTEDT

Max Planck Institute for Social Anthropology

Further Reading

Beers, Susan-Jane (2001). *Jamu: The ancient Indonesian art of herbal healing.* Tokyo, Rutland (Vermont), and Singapore: Tuttle Publishing.

Bruijn, J. R. & Gaastra, F. S. (1993). *Ships, sailors and spices: East India companies and their shipping in the 16th, 17th and 18th centuries.* Amsterdam: NEHA.

Corn, C. (1998). *The scents of Eden: A narrative of the Spice Trade.* New York, Tokyo, and London: Kodansha International.

Schivelbusch, W. (1992). *Das Paradies, der Geschmack und die Vernunft: Eine Geschichte der Genußmittel* [Paradise, taste, and reason: A history of luxury foods]. Frankfurt am Main, Germany: Fischer.

Höllmann, Thomas (2010). *The land of the five flavors: A cultural history of Chinese cuisine* (Karen Margolis, Trans.). New York: Columbia University Press.

Komroff, Manuel (1926). *The travels of Marco Polo [the Venetian]* – Revised from Marsden's. translation and edited with introduction by Manuel Komroff. New York: W. W. Norton & Company, Inc.

Xinru Liu (2010). *The Silk Road in world history.* Oxford, UK: Oxford University Press.

Contributors

All contributors are listed alphabetically, followed by their affiliations. Last names are indicated by capital letters. The names of articles are in italics.

ANDERSON, E. N. University of California, Riverside
Afghan Cuisine, Chinese Cuisine, Traditional Chinese Medicine and Diet

APAHUNG, Rosarin Sang Nongthum School Cluster, Thailand
Thai Cuisine (co-author: Gerald W. FRY)

AVIELI, Nir Ben-Gurion University of the Negev
Vietnamese Cuisine

BETZ, Joachim German Institute for Global and Area Studies (GIGA)
Tea: Southeast Asia

BUELL, Paul D. University of North Georgia
Mongolian Cuisine, Tofu, Tea: East Asia (co-author: Paul VARLEY)

CWIERTKA, Katarzyna J. Leiden University
Korean Cuisine

FELIX, Mark Stephan Mahidol University, Thailand
Malaysian Cuisine

FRY, Gerald W. University of Minnesota
Thai Cuisine (co-author: Rosarin APAHUNG)

GHANOONPARVAR, M. R. University of Texas at Austin
Iranian Cuisine

GOLDSTEIN, Darra Williams College
Central Asian Cuisines

IRESON-DOOLITTLE, Carol Willamette University
Lao Cuisine (co-author: Geraldine MORENO-BLACK)

MAGAT, Margaret C. SpecPro Professional Services (SPS)
Philippine Cuisine

MORENO-BLACK, Geraldine University of Oregon
Lao Cuisine (co-author: Carol IRESON-DOOLITTLE)

NASRALLAH, Nawal Independent scholar, USA
Iraqi Cuisine

LEAF, Murray J. University of Texas at Dallas
Rice and Rice Agriculture

LEONG-SALOBIR, Cecilia University of Wollongong
Singaporean Cuisine

RAMSTEDT, Martin Max Planck Institute for Social Anthropology
Spice Trade

SRINIVAS, Tulasi Emerson College
Indian and South Asian Cuisines

WILLIAMS, Catharina Purwani
Indonesian Cuisine

WHITE, Merry Isaacs Boston University
Japanese Cuisine

YILMAZ, Emel
Turkish Cuisine

Editorial Staff

Publisher and Editor
Karen Christensen

Project Editor
Marjolijn Kaiser

Copyeditors
Olette Trouve, David Ewing, Kathy
Brock

Typesetting & Design
Amnet

IT
Rachel Christensen, Trevor Young

Image Credits

Cover (front):   Mixed rice. Photo Credit: CCo Public domain.

Cover (back):   A two-storied Turkish teapot. Photo credit: see under page 111 below.

Page 31:   A Korean stew. Photo credit: Terence l.s.m on Visualhunt / CC BY-ND.

Page 39:   A typical homemade meal from South Asia, including roti, scrambled eggs, and chickpea dal. Photo courtesy of Muray Leaf.

Page 46:   Pad Thai. Photo courtesy of Dr. Jasmin Tanariyakul, Thammasat University.

Page 62:   Vietnamese spring rolls made with rice wrappers. Photo credit: Matthew Kenwrick on Visualhunt.com / CC BY-ND.

Page 92:   Kebab. Photo credit: Mamonello on VisualHunt / CC BY.

Page 105:   Iraqi winter salad with beetroots and white beans. Photo courtesy of Nawal Nasrallah.

Page 111:   A two-storied Turkish teapot. Photo credit: quinn.anya on Visual Hunt / CC BY-SA.

Glossary

Airag: Fermented mare's milk, a favorite drink of the Mongols.

Arkhi: Mongolian word for distilled liquors, which were first popularized by the Mongols.

Ash: Thick, pottage-like dishes important in Iranian cuisine.

Ashak: A rich Afghan sauce made from Chinese chives and tomatoes.

Ayran: Turkish national drink. This non-alcoholic beverage is a diluted and salted sour yoghurt served with meals or snacks.

Bahar asfar: Iraqi yellow spice blend similar to curry powder.

Baharat: Most common spice mix in Iraqi cuisine. A brownish mix of many ingredients including cardamom, cinnamon, ginger, cloves, and allspice.

Baklava: Famous Turkish and Greek sweet pastry. The oldest existing baklava recipe is Mongolian, and the word appears to be Mongolian in derivation.

Belacan: A fermented shrimp paste that is toasted and provides a depth of flavor to curries and *sambal* (a spicy chili-pepper-based paste). It is a quintessential ingredient in Malaysian cuisine.

Bento: A variety of pre-prepared foods served in a box in Japan. Perhaps originated in the need of samurai to bring food that would keep to the battlefield. Also popular in Korea under the name *tosirak*.

Baozi: Chinese steamed stuffed buns.

Bon cha: Korean roasted barley tea.

Bulgur: Cracked wheat.

Boov: Mongolian word for flour- (grain-) based foodstuffs ranging from pastries to dumplings.

Cai: Chinese word for vegetables. In Chinese cuisine, there is a basic distinction between between *fan* (cooked grain, typically white rice) and *cai* (vegetables or any dish eaten with grain).

Canh: A clear, light soup served with most meals in Vietnamese cuisine.

Chao mein (or *chaomian*): Chinese noodles (typically wheat) boiled and then fried with vegetables and flavorings.

Chapati (chappati): South Asian unleavened flatbread usually made of whole wheat flour and cooked on a griddle.

Che: Vietnamese rice puddings or custards sold by street vendors. They can contain glutinous rice, soy beans, black beans, green beans, tapioca, lotus seeds, ginger, sesame, and sugar.

Chopsticks: Eating and cooking utensil commonly used in East Asia, consisting of two long sticks, usually made of wood, bamboo, metal, or plastic. They are called *kuazi* in Chinese, *hashi* in Japanese, and *jeotgarak* in Korean. Their origins date back to the Chinese Zhou dynasty (1045–256 BCE).

Chotkal: Korean fermented seafood. Often added to kimchi. Originated in the seventh century.

Chou doufu: "Stinky bean curd" or "stinky tofu," a fermented product with an acquired taste much loved in China and Taiwan.

Chutney: Spiced fruit- or vegetable-based preserve used as a condiment in South Asian cuisines.

Coconut: Important in Malaysia, where coconut cream features prominently in many dishes, the oil of the coconut is used for cooking, and the sap of the flower is made into unrefined palm sugar, known as *gula melaka*, which imparts a deep caramel flavor to desserts. It is also a key ingredient in the cuisine of the Philippines, where the heart of the coconut tree is considered a delicacy.

Curry: An Anglicization of the Tamil word *kari*, curries are ground spice powders originating in South Asia and used to season meat and vegetables. The oldest extant "curry" recipe, pre-chili, is found in a courtly cookbook of the Mongol Yuan dynasty. Brought to Japan via Britain as *kare raisu*.

Dairy: A very important ingredient in Central Asian and South Asian cuisines. Central Asian dairy foods include *koumiss* (slightly fermented milk), *ayran* (yoghurt mixed with water), *kaymak* (clotted cream), and *suzma* (yoghurt cheese), and Uzbek milk soups such as *shirkovok* (milk soup with pumpkin and rice). In South Asia, dairy staples include buttermilk, curds, and *ghee* (clarified butter). Dairy is little consumed in East Asia, where most adults cannot properly digest lactose.

Dal (*dahl*): South Asian dried legumes (peas, lentils, and beans). Also used to indicate dishes (soups and stews) made from these ingredients.

Dashi: The ubiquitous soup stock of Japan.

Date: A fruit available in hundreds of varieties in Iraq, where it is also used to make *dibis* (date syrup).

Dim sum: Small, savory, high-calorie snacks, usually dumplings and buns, eaten with tea. In Cantonese it is called *dim sam*, and in Mandarin *dianxin*, literally meaning "dot the heart" or idiomatically "hits the spot."

Dolma: Stuffed vegetables in Turkish cuisine. There are two kinds of *dolma*: those filled with ground meat and eaten with a yoghurt sauce, and those filled with a seasoned rice mix and cooked in olive oil. The former is a frequent main-course dish. Also known in Iranian cuisine as *dolmeh*.

Döner: Turkish kebab made by stacking layers of ground meat and sliced leg of lamb on a large upright skewer, which is slowly rotated in front of a vertical charcoal fire. As the outer layer of the meat is roasted, thin slices can be cut and served with rice pilaf.

Doufu pi (tofu skin): This tofu skin is made from the coagulated sheets that form on the top of heated soy milk. It is used in many Chinese dishes as a meat substitute.

Dumplings: Minced meat and/or chopped vegetables wrapped with a dough typically made of wheat flour. Important in East Asian and Central Asian cuisines alike. Known as *jiaozi* in China, where they are eaten steamed or in soup. Korean *mandu* dumplings are steamed, fried, or simmered in soup. Central Asian dumplings include *manty* (large steamed dumplings filled with meat or vegetables) and *chuchvara* (small boiled dumplings).

Durian: The "king of fruits," known for tasting like heaven and smelling like hell. Popular in Southeast Asia. The Thai province of Chanthaburi is famous for its durian.

Fat-tailed sheep: Animal prized in Central Asia and Mongolia for its fat, which lends intense flavor to soups.

Flatbread: Important in Central Asia, South Asia, and Northwest China. In Central Asia, where flatbreads are eaten alone or used as a plate to hold meat or vegetable stews, the most popular flatbread is *non*, a large, flat round bread pricked in a decorative pattern with a special utensil. South Asian flatbreads include *paratha*, a crispy bread with several thin layers, *chapati* (a thicker whole-wheat bread), and *thosai* (a thin pancake made from the paste of ground lentils and rice), all of which are popular in Malaysia as well. See also *nan*.

Firni: An Afghan dessert made of a milky pudding flavored with rose water and pistachios, served for special occasions.

Five Elements and Five Phases: The five elements are earth, water, wood, metal, and fire. This Chinese cosmological scheme for the classification and description of the interaction among different material phenomena is important in many Asian cuisines. In Vietnamese cuisine, the five elements are represented by rice, soup, greens, dry-cooked dishes, and fish sauce, respectively. Korean cuisine recognizes five flavors (salt, sweet, sour, hot, and bitter) and five colors (red, green, yellow, white, and black).

Gado-gado: A famous Indonesian vegetarian dish consisting of vegetables, including tomatoes, garnished with thinly sliced boiled eggs and crushed *krupuk* (prawn crackers), dressed with a peanut sauce.

Ghee: Clarified butter. Often used in South Asian cuisines.

Goji (*Lycium chinense*): A plant known as "the poor people's vitamin pill," whose leaves and berries are among the richest sources of vitamins known. Eaten solely for their nutritional value in China.

Halva: A characteristic Iraqi dessert.

Horse: A traditional food source in Central Asia. Horsemeat sausage is a Kyrgyz delicacy.

Idli: Sri Lankan steamed rice cakes.

Jamu: Spice-based natural medicines of Java.

Jiu: Chinese word for alcoholic drinks brewed from fermented grains, usually translated as "wine," but technically a beer or ale.

Kao soi: The signature dish of the Chiang Mai area of northern Thailand, it is spicy curry soup with flat egg noodles, unique to the region.

Kavurdak: Meat that has been stewed in its own fat and then stored in vessels for long keeping. It is an ancient dish of Kazakhstan and Kyrgyzstan.

Kebab (kabab): Skewered grilled meat, either in whole pieces or ground, a feature of many Central and West Asian cuisines, but originally Turkish. Uzbekistan is famous for its variety of kebabs. One of the main categories of Iranian cuisine. Also served under the name *satay* in Malaysia.

Kedgeree: South Asian (Bengali) breakfast dish consisting of steamed rice and pulses

Khoresh: Iranian stew-type dishes that are usually served over *chelo* (plain rice).

Kimbap: Sushi rolled in sheets of seaweed, a popular Korean snack.

Kimchi: Fermented vegetables. This quintessential Korean food is available in hundreds of varieties. Modern kimchi includes chili pepper and *chotkal* (fermented salted fish). Most common is *paech'u* kimchi, made from Chinese cabbage.

Koch'ujang: Chili pepper paste used to flavor a wide variety of Korean dishes.

Kotatsu: A Japanese low dining table at which one sits on the floor. A similar table is used in Korea.

Krupuk: Indonesian prawn crackers.

Kufteh: Meat or rice balls. Especially popular in Iran, but similar dishes under similar names are eaten throughout West Asia and North Africa.

Kuku: Iranian vegetable or other soufflé-type dishes.

Laap: A salad served with raw or cooked meat or fish. It is the national dish of Laos.

Lagman: A hearty soup of lamb, carrots, and noodles found throughout Central Asia.

Lamb: A *halal* food in Islam, lamb is important in the cuisines of Northwest China, Central Asia, West Asia, and South Asia.

Merienda: A Philippine afternoon snack, as simple as a mango fruit or as elaborate as pork blood stew.

Meze: Turkish dinner appetizers, consumed in small quantities at the start of a meal and traditionally intended to accompany alcoholic drinks, especially *raki*, an anise-flavored liqueur.

Millet: A grain, farmed before 8000 BCE in the Yellow River valley of North China. Thriving in dry, cool environments, it has largely been replaced by wheat in North China. In Japan, where it arrived by 300 BCE, it (and other less refined grains) has been mostly replaced by white rice.

Monosodium glutamate (MSG): A flavoring. Isolated from seaweed in Japan in the early twentieth century, it spread rapidly in Chinese cooking since the 1960s, and is deplored by traditionalists.

Nam pla: A fish sauce which provides much of the saltiness in Thai cuisine.

Nan: (Flat)Bread baked in a *tandur* or oven. In Afghanistan, the word *nan* refers to food in general. Afghan *nan* is of the Persian type: oval, rather thin, leavened, and soft but crusty.

Nước mam: A fish sauce made from fermented long-jawed anchovy. It is ubiquitous in Vietnamese cuisine and the main component of popular dipping sauces such as *nước chấm.*

Oil: Oil used in Asian cooking comes from a wide range of plants, nuts, and seeds, including sunflower, peanuts, sesame, soy, maize, rapeseed, etc. It is used for (stir)frying and also to make dressings and sauces, and added to soups and stews.

Paan: Betel leaf and nut. Chewed as a digestive in South Asia.

Pad Thai: A dried noodle dish, the signature dish of Thai cuisine.

Panch'an: The side dishes essential to a Korean meal. The number served per meal varies. Stews (*jjigae*) and greens (blanched or sautéed and then mixed with a dressing) constitute the majority of panch'an.

Papad (*papadum*): South Asian lentil wafer, usually made from black gram flour.

Phở: Flat rice noodles in either beef broth or chicken broth with small amounts of meat. It is the most popular Vietnamese street food dish.

Pialy: A bowl-like teacup without a handle, used for ritual hospitality in Central Asia.

Pilaf: The preferred style of rice in West Asian, and later Central and South Asian cuisines. Stir-fried before boiling, pilaf contrasts with the Chinese and East Asian style, in which rice is boiled, dried, and *then* stir-fried.

Polo: Iranian rice mixed with other ingredients such as legumes, meats, vegetables, and herbs.

Pork: Important in East and Southeast Asian cuisines. The most common meat in China, which is home to two-thirds of the world's domesticated pigs.

Prasadam: Centuries-old, sophisticated, and elaborate Indian ritual food for sacred offerings to temple deities and for life-cycle rituals of devotees.

Pu'er: One of the most famous varieties of tea. It comes from Yunnan Province in China and is often sold in small prepared doses called "camel pellets."

Pulutan: Philippine snacks consumed either as street food or during drinking sessions. Believed to be a male aphrodisiac.

Puri (*poori*): Indian fried, unleavened bread, usually eaten for breakfast or with a light meal (see *thali*).

Qurt: Dried skim milk, resulting through a variety of preparations in a hard, chewy cake of low-fat milk solids. *Qurt,* a Turkic word, is commonly eaten in Afghanistan and other Central Asian countries.

Rempah: A paste made of ground herbs and spices often used in the cooking of Eurasian Singaporeans. A unique combination of European and Asian influences.

Rendang (or *Rending*): An Indonesian curry simmered in spices, chilies, and coconut until dry. Originating in West Sumatra, it is well known internationally.

Rice: Chinese *fan,* Japanese *gohan,* Korean *bab,* Vietnamese *cơm.* The rice species *Oryza sativa* is cultivated in Asia. Subspecies *japonica*, with short, fat, sticky grains, is central to the cuisines of East and Southeast Asia, where the respective languages' words for "cooked rice" refer to food generally. Subspecies *indica*, with long, thin grains, has a somewhat lesser though nonetheless great importance in South Asian cuisines.

Rice porridge (or congee): Common throughout East Asia. Called *cháo* in Vietnam, where it is made with chicken, fish, pork, shrimp, organ meat, or eel.

Rice alcohol (wine): A variety of distilled or un-distilled alcoholic beverages from Mongolia and East Asia.

Rijsttafel: An internationally acclaimed Dutch adaptation of the Indonesian feast during the festival of Lebaran at the end of Ramadan. Consists of a variety of fried dishes, curries, omelets, and greens.

Rosogollas: Bangladeshi cottage-cheese sweets

Rượu gạo: Vietnamese distilled rice alcohol. Previously the most popular alcoholic beverage in Vietnam, it has now been supplanted by beer.

Satay: Cubed, marinated meat (usually chicken) on a skewer.

Sambal: A spicy chili-pepper-based paste, popular in Indonesian and Malaysian cuisines.

Sambol (*Sambhal*): Rich coconut sauce which typifies Sri Lankan cuisine.

Sangkhaya: A traditional Thai sweet, it is a custard made from Thai tapioca.

Shülen: Banquet soups which typified the courtly cuisine of the Mongol Yuan dynasty, consisting of lamb, spices, and various ingredients. Present-day versions include ingredients as unexpected as French fries.

Sichuan pepper: Actually a prickly ash or *fagara, Zanthoxylum spp.*, traditionally used to add heat to the spicy cuisines of Sichuan and other provinces in southwest China. Now largely replaced by chilies.

Sinigang: A broth of fish or shrimp paired with vegetables and flavored with tamarind, guava, or citrus fruits. The dish represents the typical sour-salty flavor of Philippine cuisine.

Soju: The national liquor of Korea, descended from Mongolian *arkhi*.

Soy: Consumed as tofu, soy milk, soy sauce, and in other forms, soy is an important protein source in East Asia and Vietnam.

Spring roll: A wrapped appetizer. In the Philippines, *lumpia* is a fried or fresh spring roll. In Vietnam, *gỏi cuốn* are spring rolls made with rice "paper" wrappers, stuffed with greens and meat or seafood.

Sticky rice: *Oryza sativa* var. *glutinosa* (*khao niaw* in Lao), a sub-species which contains a large amount of amylopectin starch, which causes the kernels to disintegrate when boiled. So significant to the Lao that they consider it the essence of their identity.

Sushi: Actually not regularly eaten in Japan, where it is a celebratory food or special treat. Originally from Southeast Asia—not Japan. The earliest form was fermented.

Suutei tsay (*tsai*): Mongolian tea made by boiling compressed bricks of tea in milk for a long period of time, with various additives, including butter or cream.

Tandoor (*tandur*): A clay oven used to bake flatbreads in South Asia. Also important in Central Asia, where it is called *tandyr*.

Tea: *Camellia sinensis*, native to China, is the object of a vast worldwide trade. It is produced in three main varieties: as orthodox tea (the main producer is Sri Lanka), as CTC-tea (where the leaf is cut, torn, and curled before firing/heating; the main producers are India and Kenya), and as green tea (manufactured without firing; the main producer is China).

Tea Ceremony: Japanese *chado*, an art first developed in the Kamakura Period (1185–1333) by Buddhist priests. In the Edo or Tokugawa period (1600/1603–1868), the attached cuisine, *cha kaiseki ryori*, became an elaborate formal meal characterized by fresh, seasonal, high-quality ingredients.

Thali: Traditional South Asian meal, originally served on a leaf but now on a stainless steel platter, consisting of vegetable dishes, rice, *puri* or chapati (breads), pickles, lentil wafers (*papad*), yoghurt, and dessert.

Tofu: Soybean curd (Chinese *doufu*, Japanese *tofu*, Korean *tubu*, Vietnamese *dau hu*). Important in the cuisines of East Asia and Vietnam.

Tom yang kung: Lemongrass shrimp soup, a signature dish of Thai cuisine.

Tsampa: Mongolian buttered, ground grain. *Tsamba* in Tibet, where it is added, with yak butter, to tea.

Tuak: An Indonesian fermented palm wine drunk on special occasions.

Turkish delight: *Lokum* in Turkish. A jelly sweet often mixed with walnuts or pistachios, cut into cubes, and rolled in powdered sugar.

Vinegar: Made from fermented grains, vinegar is used in a number of Asian cuisines, but is most characteristic of the food of Shanxi Province, China.

Ya nang: A leaf commonly used in Lao cuisine. It is soaked and squeezed to produce a viscous green liquid added to many dishes.

Yaoshan: Chinese "medical dining" or traditional medicinal dishes. *Yaoshan* restaurants have become popular since the 1980s.

Yin and yang: An ancient Chinese cosmological principle of polar contrast and balance, integral to the cuisines and medicinal systems in East Asia. In Vietnamese cuisine, yin and yang correspond to "cold" and "hot" ingredients, respectively.

Index

Bold entries and page numbers denote main articles.

Bold entries and page numbers denote main articles.

www.ingramcontent.com/pod-product-compliance
Lightning Source LLC
Chambersburg PA
CBHW080424270326
41929CB00018B/3150

* 9 7 8 1 6 1 4 7 2 0 3 0 0 *